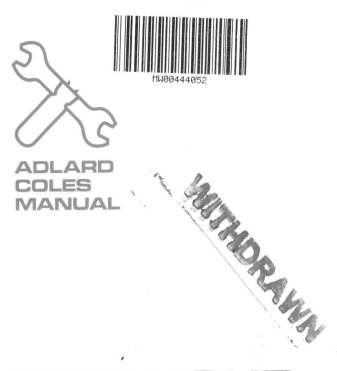

ADLARD
COLES
MANUAL

REPLACING YOUR BOAT'S ENGINE

MIKE WESTIN
Edited by John Mardall

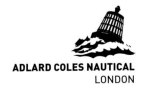

ADLARD COLES NAUTICAL
LONDON

Published by Adlard Coles Nautical
an imprint of Bloomsbury Publishing Plc
36 Soho Square, London, W1D 3QY
www.adlardcoles.com

Copyright © Michael Westin 2011.
First published in Sweden by Columbus Förlag and Praktiskt
Båtägande.
Published in the UK in 2011 by Adlard Coles Nautical.

ISBN 978-1-4081-3294-4

A CIP catalogue record for this book is available from the
British Library.

This book is produced using paper that is made from
wood grown in managed, sustainable forests. It is natural,
renewable and recyclable. The logging and manufacturing
processes conform to the environmental regulations of the
country of origin.

Typeset in URWGrotesk by James Watson.
Printed and bound in China by C&C Offset Printing Co.

Note: While all reasonable care has been taken in
the publication of this book, the publisher takes no
responsibility for the use of the methods or products
described in this book.

The author wishes to thank Jonas Arvidsson for the
illustrations aswell as the following contributors: Rolf
Ellnebrand, Kerstin Hanson, Jarle Karlsrud, Ingegerd
Lindén, Bo Linderholm, Lars Lundbladh, Kim Rask, Hans
Svedberg, Jan-G Westin, Jörgen Westin, Michael Ån and a
special thanks to the boat owners that showed me their new
installations.

>> CONTENTS

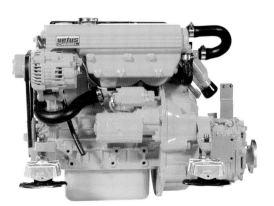

>> REPLACING A BOAT'S ENGINE

Before starting the engine replacement on my boat *Roobarb*, I wasn't sure I'd be able to pull off such a complicated and technically advanced repower and refit project. Working with a hammer and saw was not a problem, nor was making small repairs with epoxy resin and fibreglass but anything connected to electricity and engines had always filled me with dread.

I decided that it was best to jump in at the deep end – if you don't have a go, you never know what you can accomplish, and I was prepared to learn! I consider myself only an average boat owner with some basic skills when it comes to practical matters – I may not have two left hands but it's not far off. And like most, I enjoy messing around and fixing things on the boat but don't always know the best way to go about it.

The hardest thing about replacing the engine was the planning and worrying – thinking through each stage of the job, and making decisions about how to do it. Most of the time, actually doing it was quite good fun.

There were of course moments when I wondered if I should ever have started at all but these moments didn't last long, and I now have a boat with a new engine and some useful information to share with you.

PROJECT LOG

To help remember the questions I had at the beginning, I kept a log during most of the project. This proved to be very valuable while writing this book, and now that the project is complete, revisiting those early ideas and worries has been quite amusing.

I also kept a record of everything I bought so that I would know almost exactly how much the engine swap had cost me. In addition to the engine and related equipment, I felt that I had to buy some new tools even though I would be able to borrow some of the special tools that I'd only need once. In the penultimate chapter of the book, I calculate the costs that resulted directly from the replacement of the engine.

Here are some of the factors I considered before starting:

ENGINE SPECIFICATION

Beyond the purchase price of the engine, there are many questions that need to be answered before you make your final decision. You have to interpret and understand the specifications – for example, you may know about power, but what is torque and why does it matter? What reduction ratio is needed on the gearbox? Does the new engine-gearbox combination need a new propeller? Is engine weight going to be a factor? How does one engine compare with another when installed on this particular boat?

I didn't want to have to rebuild the engine bed too much, so finding an engine that would drop onto the existing bed, with minimum re-work, was also an important factor for me.

COST

No one wants to pay more than they have to for an engine or anything else, but it's important to check out the availability and price of spare parts – there's no point in buying a cheap engine and then discovering that it can't be maintained and serviced at a reasonable cost. In choosing an engine, I looked at the overall price, including the cost of spare parts and items needed for routine maintenance.

THE SCOPE OF THE PROJECT

I assumed that most of the equipment related to *Roobarb*'s engine would also need to be replaced in the repower project. I had to consider replacing the stuffing box, exhaust system, bilge pumps, fuel tanks, propeller shaft and propeller. It's better, and ultimately less expensive, to do a thorough job from the beginning, and you avoid the frustration of another period of time when your boat is out of action.

I planned to do the work in the evenings after my full-time job and on weekends. I reckoned it would take me ten weeks to carry out the tasks that had to be completed before the boat could go back in the water. Some small items could be completed after that.

I'll refer back to the project log throughout this book, to review my concerns and worries before each part of the repower and refit, and will review those issues in Chapter 8.

Changing the engine took about 300 hours in total, but a lot of that was spent in thinking through how to do the next stage. If I ever have to replace another engine, I think I'll be able to do it in about half the time that this one took.

I realise that no two boats are exactly alike and that you and I are unlikely to have exactly the same questions and concerns while replacing an engine, but I do hope you will find some of the information in this book useful.

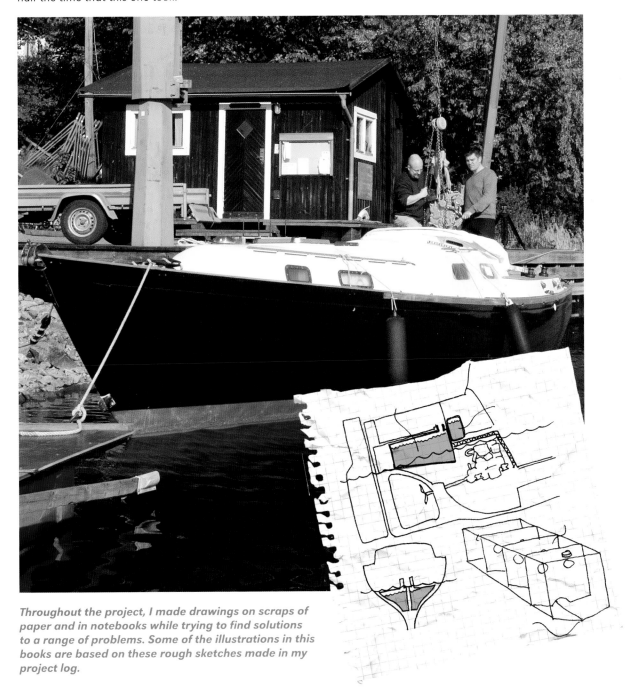

Throughout the project, I made drawings on scraps of paper and in notebooks while trying to find solutions to a range of problems. Some of the illustrations in this books are based on these rough sketches made in my project log.

›› *ROOBARB*, THE PROJECT BOAT

Americans call this type of small, long-distance boat a 'pocket-cruiser', and it was in the US that the first Vancouver 27 was constructed at the end of the 1960s by Rob Harris. Rob's clients were a couple who wanted to sail from Canada to New Zealand.

The boat's performance and sea-kindly character exceeded expectations, and series production started a couple of years later. Approximately 250 of the 27s have been produced, both in the US and England. A small change was made to the design in 1983 and another 60 of the resulting Vancouver 28s have been produced since then, with the moulds still kept at the Northshore boatyard in Itchenor.

Roobarb was built from a kit in 1977 (hull #7 in the UK). I purchased her 25 years later, to be used as the subject for many practical projects that were described in articles in the Swedish magazine *Practical Boat Owning*. Although this type of boat is not very common in Sweden, *Roobarb* displayed many of the problems that affect similar boats built in the 1970s. Indeed she has served well as the case study for a refit and improvement project that has so far included everything from reworking the teak deck to building a completely new galley.

One of the aims of the project was to make the boat ready for a long-distance cruise, and then take her on it, showing that you can go a long way, even with a limited budget.

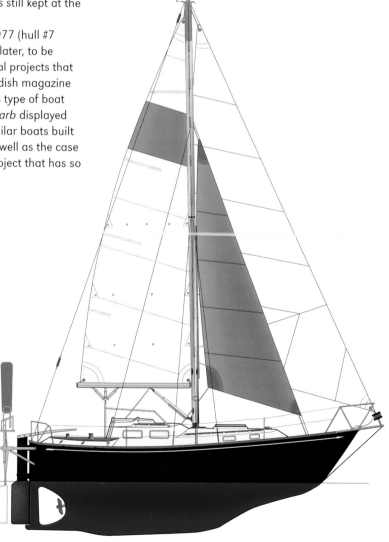

Roobarb

Length: *8.23 m*

LWL: *6.99 m*

Beam: *2.64 m*

Draught: *1.30 m*

Displacement: *approx 4.1 metric tonnes/9,039 pounds*

In the keel: *1.6 metric tonnes/3,527 pounds of lead*

Sail area: *35.2 square meters/378 square feet*

Engine: *Vetus M3.28 27.2 hp*

Fuel: *245 litres/64.7 US gallons*

01
A NEW OR REBUILT ENGINE?

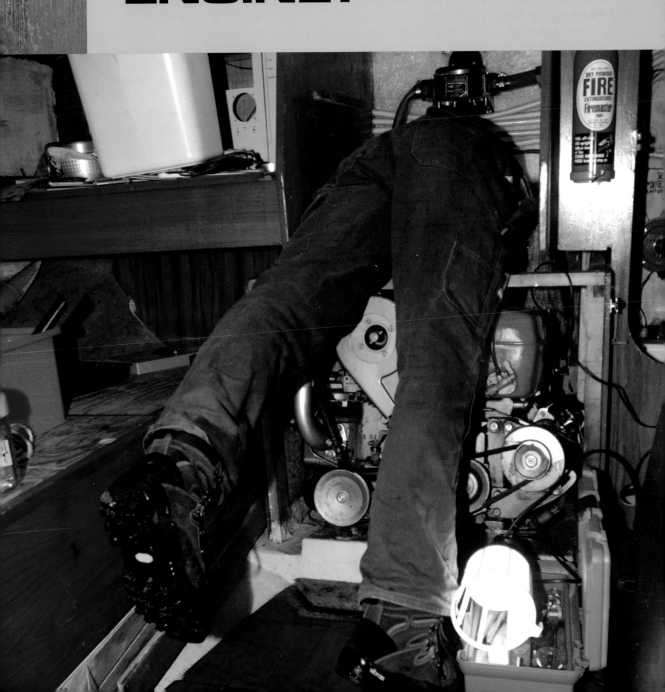

›› THE FIRST STEPS

The author's project was to replace the engine on his boat _Roobarb_. This book, however, will start from the very beginning – the process of deciding whether to rebuild the existing engine or buy a new one..

Thousands of inboard engines in the recreational fleet are approaching the end of their lives and will soon need to be rebuilt or replaced. If you are handy and able to do the job yourself, you can save a lot of money.

When your existing engine is worn out, does it make sense to rebuild it or are you better off buying a new one? Which questions do you need to answer before you decide and get started?

I have just swopped the engine in a boat for the first time. The fact is that I had never before done anything remotely similar!

However, since I consider myself to be a reasonably practical guy, I hope that what I learned from this project may be of help to other boat owners who would like to replace their own engines – without having to make the same mistakes that I made.

Since I had no previous experience, I first first tried to identify the parts of the project for which I would need guidance and technical input. I also enlisted the help of an expert. a mechanic from the local engine shop who gave me valuable advice on how to go about this job and also lent me a jig for the engine. This jig made the construction of the new engine bed much simpler, which I will show later in the book. In fact, his support and the availability of the jig were deciding factors in the final selection of a new engine.

But let's start from the very beginning when the idea of replacing the engine occurred to me. This happened when I realised that the old engine probably wouldn't last for as long as I was hoping to keep the boat...

THE ENGINE'S LIFE EXPECTANCY

An inboard marine diesel engine normally lasts between 15 and 20 years. The old Yanmar YSE12 inboard engine aboard _Roobarb_ was almost 30 years old and was beginning to show its age – unable to hold a steady speed (possibly due to a worn regulator spider in the injection pump) and needing a light hand on the two control levers to avoid stalling.

The previous owner, who had completely assembled the boat from a kit, reported using the engine sparingly – less than 500 hours in 25 years. He was a die-hard sailor and only used the engine to go in and out of the harbours he visited.

The old engine was raw water cooled, with no heat exchanger, but had been used almost exclusively in the bay of Bothnia, Sweden, where the salt content is nearly zero.

One of the main factors affecting the lifespan of old engines is corrosion from within. Many of these Yanmar engines have had a heat exchanger cooling system added at some time after the initial installation but that was not the case with _Roobarb_.

5 OPTIONS

1. **Keep going until the old engine dies**
2. **Rebuild the old engine**
3. **Buy a second-hand rebuilt engine of the same type**
4. **Buy an outboard engine**
5. **Buy a new inboard engine**

SHOULD YOU REBUILD?

The obvious alternative to buying a completely new engine is to rebuild the one you already have. It is a definite possibility if you possess the technical know-how and have some experience (yourself or someone in your circle of friends).

Getting an engine installer do the job is likely to cost a lot of money – a rough estimate could be anywhere between £1000 and £4000 for a rebuild, depending on how much you can do yourself and the condition of the engine. Add to this any spare parts and you are looking at several thousand pounds. It could end up being almost as expensive as buying a new engine. There is also the risk that a rebuilt engine will soon need to be rebuilt again.

In my case, I decided that it would be better for my long term finances and peace of mind to change to a new engine with better reliability and improved performance. Some boat owners prefer to install an outboard on a boat like this, instead of spending the money on a new or renovated inboard engine. That's understandable when you see the range of costs connected to these options.

FINDING THE RIGHT ENGINE

If you have decided to invest in a new engine rather than letting the old one keep going for another few seasons, or maybe rebuilding it, the task begins of determining which engine is most suitable for you and your boat.

The engine is only one part of the equation and you have to reckon on spending at least another £1500 for related equipment. That is if you don't want to keep the stuff that's already there and is probably as or more worn-out and trouble-prone than the old engine.

An engine installer will quote around £1500 in labour for changing an engine of this size without changing the related equipment. The engine alone for a sailing boat can cost anything from £4000 to £10,000, depending on the size and type. For a large power boat, the cost will be considerably higher.

Whichever way you look at it, changing the engine on an old boat costs a lot of money, so you need to do your research and also decide what additional equipment you should replace while the engine is out and the engine space is accessible.

GATHERING THE FACTS

My first action after deciding to buy a new engine instead of rebuilding the old one was to do some thorough research. I started searching online for information about engine replacement and I found some, but not as much as I'd expected. I also had been hoping to find a book with basic facts that described the different steps in changing an engine which would have saved a lot of head-scratching and worrying (which, of course, is the reason for writing this book).

Finally, after gathering some basic information and making a long list of questions and issues, I went to a major boat show, looking for answers and help. I spent two days at that show, investigating the market and talking to manufacturers and their dealers. In addition to being a great opportunity to talk with a lot of knowledgeable people, a boat show can also be a good place to actually buy an engine – as many manufacturers offer some kind of discount, for sales completed while the show is in progress.

ADDITIONAL FACTORS

It shouldn't only be the price that determines your choice of engine. Many boats have a very tight engine space, under the companion way stair or cockpit, and service points such as dip sticks, filters, pump housings and oil fills and coolant fills all need to be easily accessible without having to remove parts of the boat's interior. The size of the engine and the location of filters and other components also need a lot of thought.

Older engines often revolve more slowly than their modern engines counterparts, making it difficult to keep the same stern gear and propellers. There

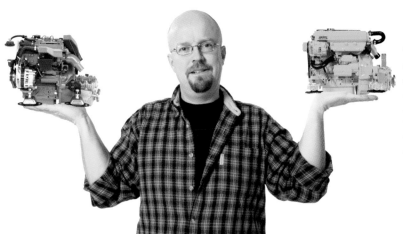

To choose an engine is not the easiest of tasks. Different brands have different advantages and no engine has it all. As usual, there have to be compromises. In Chapter 9 I've put together a guide to the most common (and some less common) inboard engines on the market – a summary that would have helped when I was looking for an engine myself.

are adapter kits available but it might be worth considering changing the whole drive train as a part of the repower project – sometimes you don't have a choice, the shaft and prop have to be replaced.   As an added complication the new engine may rotate in the other direction, and depending on the type of gearbox, that may make a new propeller a necessity.

ENGINE OUTPUT

All the engine dealers with whom I spoke recommended engines for *Roobarb* in the 20–30 horse powerrange (15–22 kilowatt). Several of them suggested an output of around 25 horse power. The recommendations varied a bit, depending on the sizes of engine offered by each manufacturer.

One sales rep suggested that the boat could use around 40 horsepower to push it through rough seas. It's true that there will be times when you wish you had a more powerful engine, but bigger also mean more expensive to buy, service and operate.

If I followed the rule-of-thumb formula of 4-5 horse power per metric tonne of boat (5 tonnes with the boat loaded for a longer trip) the power requirement for *Roobarb* should be somewhere between 20–25 horse power (approx. 15–18 kilowatt).

I thought it made sense to go to the upper end of the range, especially as of the more powerful engines I looked at, almost all weighed less than the 140 kilograms of the old Yanmar.

The boat was going to go from a one cylinder engine to a three cylinder one, with three times more power. It would probably run more smoothly, and be better for the environment. I assumed that the fuel consumption of the new engine would be marginally higher than for the old one. The fuel consumption of the old Yanmar YSE12 was approximately one litre per hour at around 1200 rpm with a boatspeed of 4.5–5 knots

TORQUE

One of the arguments I heard at the show was that the torque is better on new engines than on older generation models with similar horsepower. Torque and output go hand in hand, but torque is less related to boat speed than to the engine's ability to push the boat against a strong headwind or through a heavy chop.

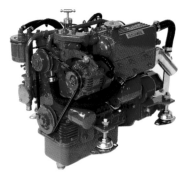

The Beta Marine 25 horsepower engine is ideal in that it has all the important service points collected at the front of the engine within easy reach from the under-the-companionway stairs in the cabin.

Read more in the fact box on page 5 about how to interpret the manufacturers' brochures.

SIZE

If the engine space on your boat is small, the dimensions of the new engine you select become critical. Common concerns also include how the oil sump protrude under the engine and if the engine and gearbox can be installed low enough to fit onto the propeller shaft.

All the service points must also be easily accessible. Some engines are set up to allow the pumps and filters to be unbolted from the engine and remotely mounted on a bulkhead or other surface in the engine room, or even outside it.

You have the boat you have, and you probably don't want to rebuild it to take a bigger engine. With a little bit of planning (and maybe a lightweight mock-up of the new engine) you can figure out whether a particular engine will fit or not.

In the next chapter we will take a look at the dimensions and construction of the all-important engine bed.

THE FINAL CHOICE

All of the engines I considered had their special features and none of them seemed to be a bad choice. Several dealers confirmed that there few significant differences between modern engines. It is more likely to be related issues that tip the balance in choosing an engine; such as being able to get help with the installation (if you need help) near where you intend to do the work.

Or perhaps you need an engine that is compatible with an existing item of equipment such as an S drive transmission (Volvo 110, 120, etc.) that you want to keep on the boat.

The deciding factors in my choice of a 27 horse power three cylinder Mitsubishi engine marinized by Dutch firm Vetus den Ouden, was that I could borrow a jig – a frame model of the engine – to facilitate construction of the new engine bed – and that I had access to sound advice form a Vetus dealer close to the boat club where *Roobarb* is moored.

The purchase price of the Vetus engine was also a good deal, as I bought one that had been at a boat show. The fact that Vetus could supply a lot of the additional equipment that I would need contributed to my decision. Not having to chase around town looking for equipment would be a benefit – although in the end there was to be a fair amount of running around anyway.

Whether or not I will be able to find the necessary spare parts in the far-flung places I hope to visit with *Roobarb* remains to be seen. The people at Vetus have told me that in addition to having dealers in many parts of the world, they routinely air-freight spare parts to boats in very remote locations – it's a part of the reality of customer support and service in the boat equipment business.

The old Yanmar engine was eventually sold on the Internet for £600 to someone who had the knowledge and inclination to rebuild the engine.

BEFORE THE START

Before the physical work started and also during the project, I kept a log in order to later remember where I had problems and to describe them in writing. I also kept a record of everything I bought so that I would know almost exactly how much the engine swop had cost me.

In addition to the engine and related equipment, I felt that I had to buy some new tools even though I would be able to borrow some of the special tools that I'd only need once.

In the penultimate chapter of the book, I calculate the costs that resulted directly from the replacement of the engine.

Units of measurement

Horsepower:
In many English-speaking countries, engine output is measured in horsepower, while much of the rest of the world uses kilowatts.

To convert	to	Multiply by
kilowatt	horsepower	1.341
horsepower	kilowatt	0.746
metric horsepower	horsepower	0.9863
litres	gallon (UK)	0.21997
litres	gallon (US)	0.26417
gallons (UK)	litres	4.546
gallons (US)	litres	3.785
gallons (US)	gallons (UK)	0.83268
gallons (UK)	gallons (US)	1.20094
ton (UK)	tonnes (metric)	1.016

To convert fuel consumption in MPG (miles per gallon) to l/100km (litres per 100 kilometres) divide 282.5 by the MPG figure.

FOCUS | DISADVANTAGES OF OLD ENGINES

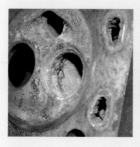 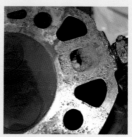

These coolant channels on an old Yanmar YSE12 which are blocked around the cylinder walls. The coolant channels in the cylinder head have corroded all the way through and into the cylinder.

It costs a lot of money to rebuild an engine that is 20–30 years old and it's probably not money well spent unless you can do the rebuild yourself, and save the labour costs. It may be worth it on a late model engine that will keep running for several more years, but think carefully – this is not an easy job, and you can't know what you'll need to replace until you open up the old engine. You may be deep into a rebuild, in time and money, when you discover that something is broken that can't be replaced, and then all the work you've done and all the money you've spent are down the drain.

COMMON PROBLEMS WITH OLD ENGINES

- Older engines frequently don't have fresh water cooling, and the cooling channels in the block and cylinder head may have corroded or be blocked by sediment and rust. In order to inspect the condition of the channels, the cylinder head must be removed.
- The rubber in the engine mounts has lost all of its elasticity and the mounts have collapsed, so that the engine and gearbox are no longer aligned with the propeller shaft. Most manufacturers recommend changing the engine mounts every 5–7 years.
- The exhaust mixing elbow is exposed to a lot of hot exhaust gas and corrosive salt water, and is among the first things to go. Having said that, it's not too hard to replace a mixing elbow if a new one is still available.

- Not all old engines have exchangeable oil filters. Sometimes they have a permanent filter on a screw-threaded mount and these have to be taken out regularly and cleaned in paraffin/ kerosene.
- Fuel filters are not common on older engines, which may mean that dirt has penetrated the engine. The cylinders may have been so worn that grooves and ridges exist on the cylinder walls. The cylinders will need to be rebored and honed and new, larger pistons and piston rings will need to be installed. For larger engines with removable cylinder walls, known as 'wet sleeves', it's sometimes possible to replace the sleeves as well as the pistons and rings, so reboring and honing is not required, but don't expect any of this to be easy.
- The cylinder head corrodes through and is expensive or impossible to replace. New replacement heads are rarely available and second-hand ones of good quality are hard to find. To detect this problem the cylinder head has to be removed for inspection.
- The high-pressure fuel pump spider may be caked in carbon soot or blocked by dirt and debris. Unstable speed is a common problem with YSE-engines. The cause may be a worn-out regulator spindle on the injection pump.
- Hoses and seals on copper pipes and fittings have dried out and become brittle. These parts should be changed every 5–10 years.

What do the experts say?

I asked the retailers at the boat show if they had any tips for people thinking of replacing the engine themselves; including what other jobs one might do at the same time and what power output they recommended for the project boat *Roobarb*. Together, these four people I quote below have more than 100 years of experience with the replacement of boat engines..

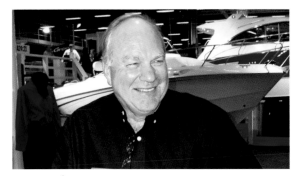

Lennart Åkerberg works at Soberg Marine and has serviced, installed and sold boat engines and run engine workshops for more than 43 years. Soberg Marine sells Yanmar and Beta engines.

THE EXPERT: 'IF IN DOUBT – DO IT NOW'

In Lennart Åkerberg's opinion, the first thing to think about when changing to a new engine is to make sure that the new engine fits in the engine space. Check where the service points will be so that fuel filters, oil filters and the more water pump impeller are all easy to reach and replace. There must also be room above the engine to adjust valve clearances and refill oil and coolant. It's often to do some minor re-working of the engine space to make service points accessible.

As Lennart said, if more than minor adjustments are required for a particular engine, think twice about it – you may have to make some major interior changes to the boat, with many unforeseen consequences involving a lot of work you hadn't planned on doing.

Lennart talked about how he has to saw in to some modern boats to repair or replace an engine, or in extreme cases even to perform the boat builder's own recommended maintenance procedures. 'Not so good', said Lennart, with some irony in his voice.

Lennart also warned that the engine beds on some older boats can be in very poor condition; and may even have completely detached from the hull and will require repairs.

It is no longer possible to buy ready-made engine beds but you can easily make your own with a pair of flat steel bars that can be drilled and threaded for the engine mounts. There are still special engine beds available for boats with saildrives; for which a special beds are usually essential.

MORE TO THINK ABOUT

Something else that must be done while the engine is out of the boat is to check, and probably replace, the propeller shaft seal, shaft bearing(s), engine controls, and control cables, says Lennart.

Lennart also recommended that I should also put in new fuel/water separating filters or at least replace the elements of the existing fuel filters. And you must check that the fuel hoses, coolant hoses, seacocks, skin fittings and through-hulls are in good condition. Don't forget, the difficulty and cost of replacing any of these items goes up dramatically after the new engine is installed. If in doubt – do it now. The accessories excluding the engine itself normally cost around £1500, says Lennart.

THE RECOMMENDATION FOR *ROOBARB*

For *Roobarb*, Lennart recommended Yanmar's 22 horsepower diesel, or possibly their 29 horsepower three cylinder diesel engine. He said that the larger engine would make it easier for the boat to push through big seas and fight strong currents. Lennart also reminded me that a three cylinder engine runs more smoothly and quietly than the single cylinder unit I was replacing.

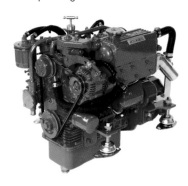

THE EXPERT: 'CONSIDER ALL SMALL JOBS TO ESTIMATE THE COST'

Mats started his remarks with a very basic but fundamentally important question, that it is easy to overlook as you get embroiled in the details of an interesting and complicated project: Before you start replacing the engine, which is a very big financial commitment, do you really like this boat and intend to keep it?

There are many things you need to think about replacing, such as the fuel system. The electrical system also needs to be inspected carefully; because a new engine often has a much bigger alternator that may require larger charging cables.

Mats gave some good advice about what to think about a new propeller; the propeller shaft seals almost always need replacing. That also goes for the propeller since the reduction ratios of the new gearbox and the direction of rotation almost always differ from the old one.

In order to calculate the correct propeller dimensions, Mats uses a computer program (Volvo Penta's Marine Propulsion System) into which he enters the measurements of the boat, its weight and the type of hull, so that the program can work out the correct propeller type, diameter and pitch. After this, Mats explores different data to find the best possible combination of propeller and range of boat speed. A propeller with a small diameter but large pitch allows a higher top boat speed to be reached. However a large diameter prop with moderate pitch, rotating more slowly, can better harness the torque of the engine for a more powerful push at low and moderate boat speeds against breaking waves, chop and current.

COSTS

Mats estimated that supplemental equipment costing approximately £1500 would be added to the cost of the engine itself. In addition, the labour cost for replacing the engine, which normally takes 40–45 man hours on a boat like this, would total about £2500 including VAT.

When you use a professional installer you must expect to pay for any additional work or services you require that are not in the quote, so analyze your project carefully and read the quote carefully.

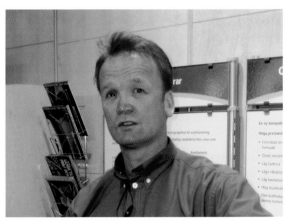

Mats Lindström works at Lindströms Wharf in Dalarö, Sweden mainly on power boat renovations involving the installation of new engines. The company sells and services Volvo Penta equipment.

For example sound insulation for the engine room is offered separately by Lindströms Wharf, since it is a job not required on some boats and it can take a lot of time.

Mats usually reckons on 5–6 man hours to remove the old sound insulation and cut and glue the new panels. All in all, the replacement of an engine will cost at least £8000, depending on which engine you choose and if you can get a good discount when you buy it.

Mats agreed with me that it's a lot of money, but worth it if you're going to keep and enjoy the boat. Mats went on to say: 'You have to distinguish between expensive and a lot of money. Something becomes expensive when you don't think it's worth the money. With a new engine, the boat gets a new lease of life. If you plan to keep it for another few years, it can certainly be well worth the money, especially when you consider how much a new boat will cost you.'

THE RECOMMENDATION FOR *ROOBARB*

For our project boat, *Roobarb*, Mats recommended a Volvo Penta D1-30 (28 hp) He thought that it would provide suitable power, but said that he might also consider a slightly larger engine, maybe even the 38 hp Volvo Penta D2-40, given that the boat will be heavy for its length when fully loaded.

THE EXPERT: 'CHANGE EVERYTHING WHEN YOU'RE AT IT'

Bo Linderholm's best tip was to start by doing a lot of research on what is on the market. Chat with dealers and manufacturers' reps to see what they have to offer. Bo went on to say that many old boats are under-powered, so it's important to go back to basics in deciding what size engine your boat really needs – don't just assume that the old engine has the right power output, recommended Bo. Bo said that it's also important to find an engine that fits in the engine space available, something that also applies to service points such as impeller and dipstick, etc that must be easily accessible – especially when you are in a hurry! Finding an engine that fits the space makes the repower project much easier. To be able to ascertain what needs changing and what can be reused when replacing the engine you first need to go through the whole drive train; which means engine, gearbox, couplings, propeller shaft, shaft seal, bearings and propeller.

The next things you need to check are the exhaust system, controls, and control cables (or wires in the case of electronic controls – not often found on small sailboats like *Roobarb*). Sometimes it's possible to reuse the old equipment but it has to be in excellent condition. If it isn't, replace it, recommended Bo.

Beyond that, when it comes to coolant hoses, fuel hoses and other perishable items. Bo recommends replacing them all: It's such a small amount of money in relation to the cost of the whole replacement of the engine. He added that since I have decided to undertake a job as big as replacing the engine, I may as well take the opportunity to upgrade the electrical system, even if it has no direct impact on the engine installation. There's a lot of equipment not directly related to the engine that will be affected by the repower job, and it needs to be thoroughly inspected and evaluated for replacement.

'Don't just put in a new engine and ignore the rest, it won't work' said Bo, who added that all the engines on the market are good buys and that there are many other factors that need to be considered for the whole thing to work.

'Ask if the manufacturer or dealer can offer practical help and support if you decide to do all or part of the replacement yourself', he continued.

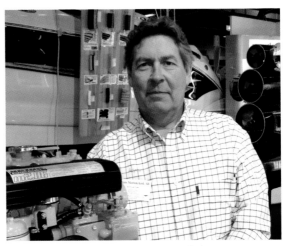

Bo Linderholm has been running Ålstens Marine Tech for 25 years. The company provides winter storage and service for recreational boats. For the last ten years Bas has sold and installed inboard diesel engines from the Dutch marine equipment company, Vetus. He has also sold Volvo Penta engines.

THE RECOMMENDATION FOR *ROOBARB*

For the project boat, Bo recommended a stronger three cylinder 28 horsepower diesel engine, since the 16 horsepower engine that was first suggested could prove to be a bit weak for such a heavy boat, especially in rough conditions ...

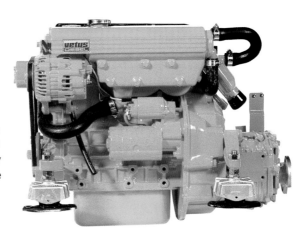

THE EXPERT: 'MAKE SURE YOU GET GOOD SUPPORT FROM THE SELLER'

Patrick Dahlgren thinks that the first step when changing an engine is to decide how much output you are going to need. Next is to determine how well the engine fits in the boat. More than this, there are only really three other areas that require extra attention; modifying the existing engine bed; orientation of the engine; and setting up a cooling water intake and exhaust system such that water cannot run back into the engine. This includes properly locating a vacuum break air vent. When it comes to additional equipment, Patrick said that the propeller almost always needs changing.

'In addition to the engine costs, you need to at least add the cost of a new propeller. Also – far too often, boats from the '70s aren't equipped with a water strainer. A new intake strainer only costs a few pounds and should be installed when replacing the engine. Most of the hoses will also need changing'.

Rohdahl Marine was founded in 1965, and imports marine engines, marine transmissions, propellers and installation accessories. Patrick Dahlgren is in the third generation of his family at Rohdahl Marine. Patrick has only been away from the company while studying to become a machine engineer and during his National Service as a machinist in the Navy.

COST

Patrick told me that the costs depend entirely on how much needs to be changed on the boat. Some people think that it is good to re-use the propeller and all of the engine-related accessories but experience leads me to plan on changing considerably more than just the engine.

'All responsible engine salesmen ask the buyer what equipment is already in the boat and will specifically list the costs for additional and necessary additional equipment in the quote. When you compare different brands of engine, it is important not only to compare price lists but also to check the trade-in price for the old engine'

I asked Patrick what problems are most commons when a novice tackles replacing an engine. Patrick told me that he usually spends a lot of time with the customer both before and after the purchase of a new engine, and always tries to determine if the customer has understood his tips and advice.

'That's why there are rarely any problems. Of course it occurs that the customer ends up in trouble for not following our advice regarding the cleaning of the fuel tank or the replacement of a fuel hose but it doesn't happen that often. We always say that it is better to phone us one time too many than one time too few'

THE RECOMMENDATION FOR *ROOBARB*

After taking into account the planned cruise and the displacement of the boat, Patrick recommended a Lombardini engine of 30 hp, and said that that engine would give *Roobarb* a real improvement in comfort and the best possible manoeuvrability. There would also be a fair amount of spare capacity, which is desirable in boats intended for a lengthy cruise. The increase in cost to go from a 20 hp Lombardini to that manufacturer's 30 hp engine was only about £450.

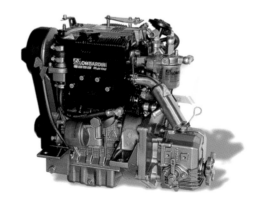

FOCUS UNDERSTANDING FUEL CONSUMPTION AND AND TORQUE

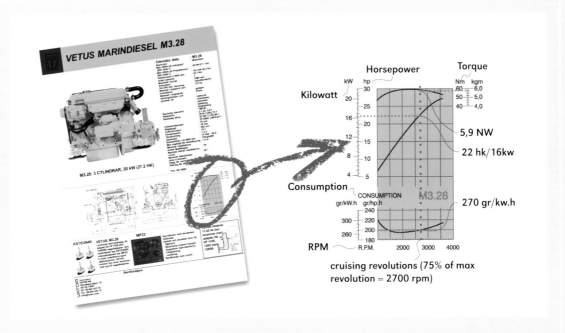

The graphs from the engine manufacturers are not always easy to interpret – and hence make it difficult to compare engines.

The catalogues, brochures and other publications from the engine manufacturers are not always easy for a lay person to understand – no two manufacturers present their numbers in the same way, and the engines can be difficult to compare.

If you lack a technical background, the different numbers can be very confusing. What do 'torque' and 'revolutions' mean and how is 'fuel consumption' interpreted?

Most people probably do as I did: they decide on the level of help and service available rather than on the technical specifications.

After taking a closer look at the documents, I still found that the different manufacturers present their numbers in ways that are difficult to compare, especially when it comes to fuel consumption.

It isn't the speed of rotation (revolutions per minute or rpms) that determines how much fuel an engine will use. The regulator on a diesel engine will keep the engine on the number of revolutions that you have set it at. The amount of fuel used at that number of revolutions is a function of the load. Factors such as the shape of the hull, how easily water flows around the hull, propeller configuration and the condition and cleanliness of the propeller all affect how much resistance the water has against the hull. These are all forms of drag, which the engine must be powerful enough to overcome in order to push the boat through the water at the maximum speed intended by the designer or naval architect.

Naval architects and boat manufacturers use a formula that includes the key dimensions of the hull to calculate the drag (or resistance to movement on the hull created by the water and

Calculation example 1

75% of the max revolutions 3,600 x 0.75 = 2,700 rpm

Achieved effect at 2,700 rpm = 16 kW/22.5 hp

Achieved fuel consumption = 270 grams/kW/h

Consumption/hour x the effect, 270 x 16 = 4,320 grams/hour

Converted to litres/hour: 4,320 x 0.00122* = 5.27 litres/hour

The engine consumes at 2,700 rpm/16kW ca 5.27 litre/hour or 1.39 US gallons per hour

* See fact box opposite for conversion factors

breaking waves or chop). The factor created in these calculations varies and is usually between 2.2 and 3.0. A rule-of-thumb factor of 2.7 is frequently used for recreational boats with displacement hulls (boats that don't plane). Some manufacturers use this factor in their calculations; others include max resistance at top boat speed. As an example of the results of this variability in calculating fuel consumption, the very safe number on the fact sheet for a Vetus M3.28 operating at full power is almost 5.3 litres per hour, whereas my experience with *Roobarb* indicates that for a sailing boat of this size and weight, motoring in flat water, 1.5 litres per hour is more realistic with this engine.

How can the published fuel consumption numbers vary so much for similar engines? It could be that the engineers at Vetus in the Netherlands use their computers to calculate consumption for maximum load, while the engineers at Volvo Penta and Yanmar assume that the boat is light in the water and thereby get numbers that correspond better to real conditions.

FUEL CONSUMPTION

Naval Architects and Engineers assume that 75% of an engine's maximum power output will be required to move the boat at its recommended cruising speed. This percentage is applied to the majority of boats powered by small inboard diesel engines. 75% output corresponds to 22.5 hp/ 16 kW for the Vetus M3.28, and on the power curve diagram in the Vetus catalogue you can read across and see that this output occurs at 2,700 rpm. To determine how much fuel the engine uses at this output, with the boat at cruising speed, you read the lower diagram for the M3.28 and can see that the consumption is 270 grams per kilowatt per hour.

Converting into litres per nautical mile (l/M) is tricky since it very much depends on the boat and conditions, but once you know what speed you typically get at cruising speed, you can work it out yourself.

The consumption according to the Vetus fact sheet for M3.28 is approx. 5.3 litres per hour (l/h)/1.4 US gallons per hour. Vetus says that it is a theoretical number for max load and the consumption from experience is about 1.5 l/hour/ 0.4 US gallons per hour. This figure is closer to the consumption given by Yanmar and Volvo for engines in the same output class.

Roobarb's tanks hold a total of 245 litres/64.7 US gallons of diesel should, so in calm conditions, I should have enough for 160 nautical miles of motoring, say from Cowes to northern Brittany, before it is time to fill up again. Long distance sailors usually calculate the range of the engine in hours or days. On *Roobarb*, the engine can run almost 32 hours at cruising speed before the tanks are empty. However, this depends partly on whether there is headwind and waves and how much fouling there is on the hull. Just as when you calculate the litres or gallons per mile for your car, you can check how much fuel you put in your boat and compare it with engine hours and average engine speed in rpm's to get a rough estimate of the fuel consumption. You can also buy a fuel flow meter if you want to track fuel consumption at different power settings.

Numbers from the manual for the vetus M3.28
Maximum output:
At flywheel (ISO 3046-1) 20 kW (27.7 hp)

On the propeller shaft (ISO 3046-1) 19.2 kW (26.2 hp)

Torque at 3,000 rpm: 53.1 Nm (39.2 ft/lbs)

Maximal revolutions: 3,600 rpm

Fuel consumption at 2,600 rpm: 270 grams/kW/h; 199 grams/hp/h

Conversion
One metric horsepower (Europe):

1 hp = 0.74 kW

1 kW = 1.36 hp

1 gram/hour = 0.00122 l/h (litre/hour, diesel has a specific weight = approx. 0.836)

Terminology
ISO 3046-1 is the European standard that describes how output and fuel consumption must be described and tested.

Torque is the turning moment of a force rotating around a point (on an engine that point is the centre of the long axis of the crankshaft). It is the result of multiplying the power by the perpendicular distance between that pivot point and the line of direction of the power, ie the lever arm or moment arm. The torque is measured in Newton meter (Nm) or foot pounds (ft/lbs). It can be described as a measure of an engine's pulling power.

The fuel consumption is normally given in grams per kilowatt per hour (g/kW x h) translated to litres per hour at cruising revolutions of 2,700 rpm (approx. 75% of the maximum revolution). However, make sure you understand to which engine speed (rpm's) the stated fuel consumption rate applies.

The standard **density of diesel** is calculated at 836 kg/m3 (the same as 836g/l) or 7.2 pounds per US gallon. Diesel has a density of 83% that of water. A tank that takes 100 litres of diesel has fuel corresponding to 84 kilo in it when it is full.

02

TAKING OUT THE OLD ENGINE

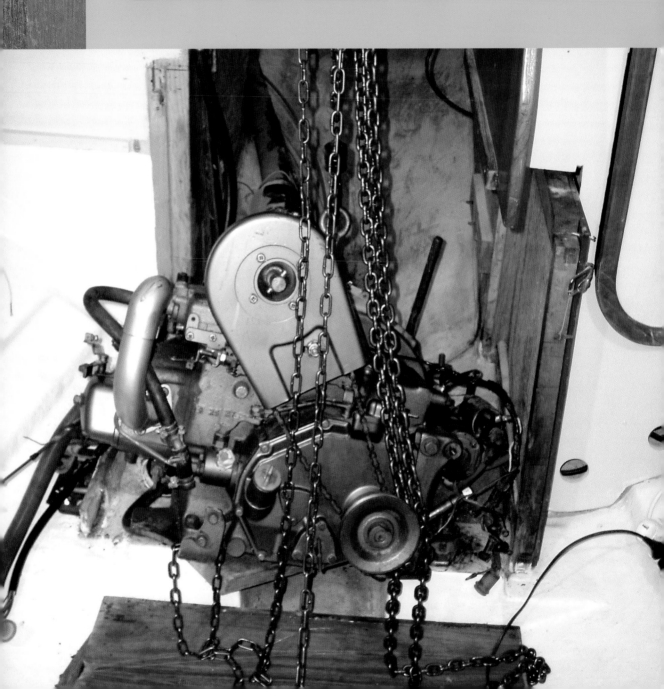

>> THE BIG LIFT

This chapter covers the difficult task of removing the old engine from *Roobarb* and the lengthy cleaning out of the engine room with its 30-year accumulation of dirt and debris.

The methods I describe here are not always the best ways of doing things. I discovered after my project that lifting out an old engine is best done with a shore-side crane or derrick while the boat is still in the water. You may learn from my mistakes!

At my sailing club's dry storage yard the boats are placed so close to each other that it was impossible to get near *Roobarb* with a mobile crane. I had to find another way of lifting out the old engine and lowering in the new one. I started by purchasing a chain hoist with one tonne capacity for about £40.

With *Roobarb*'s layout it wasn't difficult to lift the engine off the engine bed and onto a piece of scrap plywood (to protect the floorboards), so I placed a sturdy wooden beam (sawn fir) made of two 47 x 150 mm (2" x 6") beams, nailed together, with the resulting 94 mm side as the edge or bearing face resting on the cabin top over the companionway.

I used plywood spacer plates under the beam ends to raise the beam enough to protect the surround trim of the companionway hatch. I then moved the engine in small steps, raising and lowering it as we edged the beam forward, until the engine was in the cabin, directly under the hatch opening. This was the easy part!

LIFTING APPARATUS

I investigated several approaches to building a hoisting frame to lift the engine completely out of *Roobarb*, including systems of steel beams and trolleys. But in the end I used some simple steel piping of the type sold to make temporary boat tents. I braced this with wooden posts and props, and moved the engine over the cockpit, over the transom and clear of the stern by raising and lowering it while walking the chain hoist and its support props back in small steps.

Before starting this procedure, you need to have a sturdy wooden platform or board ready for the engine, so that it doesn't do any damage to the cabin sole, cockpit sole or seats. Fortunately for me,

my Uncle JG, a very practical guy, helped me with this part of the project – it's definitely not a one-man job.

The hardest part was getting the engine all the way down to a wooden pallet on the ground. My lifting frame wasn't high enough to get the engine over the stern rail, so we had to remove the rail. Then it turned out that the chain hoist did not have enough drop to get the engine all the way down to the ground, so it dangled in mid air while we rigged up another platform to hold it half-way while we lowered the chain hoist with longer straps from the ridge pole.

A Yanmar YSE12 weighs just under 140 kgs/ 308 lbs – a big chunk of heavy metal to move. Dropping an engine on your toes or your boat would definitely do a lot of damage, so it's a must to think through the lifting method before you start.

Obviously, if you can use a crane, derrick, forklift or other piece of boatyard equipment, that's the fastest and safest way to go, either while the boat is still in the water or when it's on dry land, even if that means paying for some access space, or waiting until an accessible place becomes available.

CLEANING UP & PREPARATION

When the engine space was empty, with the engine and old equipment removed, I could start cleaning it in preparation for repainting. First I blasted any loose material off with a high-pressure water machine (180 bar/2,600 psi). Then, wearing protective rubber gloves and goggles, and hanging my head down in the bilge, I used degreasing compound and plastic scourers to get at every nook and cranny. It's essential to take frequent breaks from working in this position, to avoid the blood rushing to one's head, with the danger of fainting and dropping all the way into a bilge full of caustic chemicals, dirty water, oily scum and other unhealthy substances – not a good way to go, and who wants a tombstone reading 'drowned in his own bilge'.

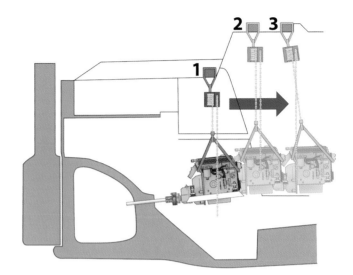

The removal of the old engine from the engine room to the plywood board on the saloon sole was completed by raising and lowering the engine, while the support beam was moved in several small steps.

Do not use steel wool for this purpose or any other onboard cleaning work – it will leave particles in the fibereglass that will bleed rust forever.

All water and debris in the bilge are vacuumed up with an industrial wet and dry vacuum cleaner. This was used frequently during the project.

The process was hard and boring but the satisfaction of a job well done was enormous, and this is not just a cosmetic issue, it's much easier to maintain and service an engine in a clean, uncluttered space.

Painting the engine space

With everything clean, I was ready to start painting. The first step in the preparations was another thorough cleaning and degreasing, but this time with paint thinner and acetone. A good extractor fan for ventilation, respiratory protective equipment, eye protection, rubber gloves and a protective disposable 'paper' suit are essential for this as with all boat painting.

Remember, modern marine coatings and their solvents can be highly toxic, some causing irreversible lung damage if inhaled when being applied by spray gun. I chose to use a two-part paint so that the finished surface would stand up to water as well as possible. After checking with the paint manufacturer's rep that the primer and topcoat were compatible with each other, I applied two coats of primer then three coats of two-part bilge paint. Even this type of paint

is not meant to be permanently submerged and can start to come off if the bilge stays wet.

In the long run, with a constantly wet bilge, there is also an increased risk of osmotic damage (the dreaded boat-pox) in which water is drawn into the fibreglass laminations of the hull, blistering the surface in the process. This is much more common on the exterior of the hull, but it can happen to the inside, with consequences including a reduction in strength and impact resistance.

Two-part paint is durable but usually requires that any old one-pack paint be removed first. Once again, if you don't want to end up with a terrible mess, check with the paint manufacturer's rep, and if in doubt, take off the old paint. On the plywood storage bins under the cockpit I used oil based (alkyd) paint that I hoped would provide a better surface for the self-adhesive sound insulation panels I intended to apply to them.

Before I could do any of this painting I had to get the surfaces not just clean but also dry, which is easier said than done in the bilge of an old boat. My preferred method is to pump (or vacuum) the bilge dry, mop up every last drop, do whatever it takes to keep water out of it, and let it dry for a couple of weeks. You have to be very thorough and patient – slapping paint on is the easy bit – any painter will tell you that success is all in the prep work.

If you do not dry out the bilge and engine spaces properly, you can be fairly certain that the new paint will peel off in patches, spoiling all your hard work.

FOCUS PAINTING WITH TWO-PART PAINT

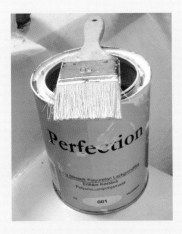

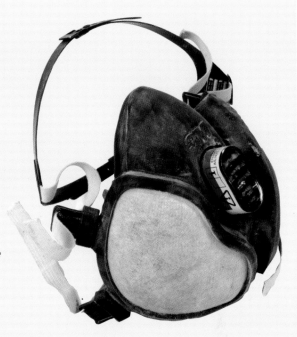

Above *All two-part paints come in two pots, the smaller of the two containing hardener.*

Right *A protective mask should be worn at all times while using polyurethane paint.*

Two-part polyurethane coatings, formulated for application in a bilge give a very hard surface that is easy to clean and fairly waterproof. The paint should not be under water permanently, but that's hard to avoid at the lowest point of the bilge. If you know that there's always going to be some water present, as occurs in most fin keel boats with a small bilge sump, follow the paint manufacturer's instructions to the letter, and consider an extra coat or two of primer (probably epoxy) before applying the two-part coating.

All two-part paints come in two pots, the smaller of the two containing hardener. The primer is applied in two to three layers with 14 to 72 hours maximum time between coats, in accordance with the paint manufacturer's recommendations. Paint in temperatures above 15 degrees Celsius/59 degrees Fahrenheit and only after thorough preparation, including sanding and washing.

As the last step, you apply one, two or better three layers of two-part bilge paint. This will give you a smooth surface that is easy to keep clean, durable and resistant to chemicals, oil and diesel.

These paints contain isocyanates which are highly toxic and potentially damaging to your airways and lungs, so be sure to use real respiratory protective equipment and protective goggles.

The paint is applied with a foam roller or a brush, in light coats. Using a brush will result in a smoother finish, if that is important to you (it's rarely necessary in an engine room). Two-part paint should never be applied onto alkyd or one-pack paint, although you can apply those paints over an existing two-part surface. Paint leftovers should go to the recycling station. Two part topside paint is ideal for painting the hull, and can sometimes be used on plastic parts in the engine room.

>> STEP-BY-STEP

To use the roof ridge (as I did) of a boat tent only works if the tent framing members are strong enough. In our case, we supported the ridge pole with wooden props set about 300mm/one foot on either side of the pulley's attachment. This meant that we had to put the engine down every other foot to reset the props. The small size of the boat tent limited our ability to construct any additional supports that might have been a better solution.

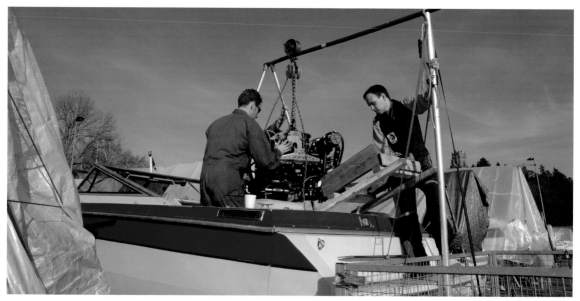

There are as many ways of removing engines as there are boat owners. The craftsmen who picked the engine out of this motor boat had constructed scaffolding that provided a straight drop into their trailer.

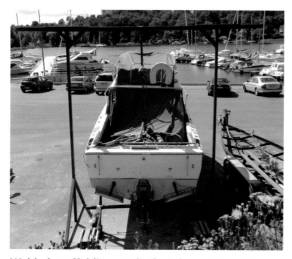

Welded scaffolding made the job considerably easier on this boat.

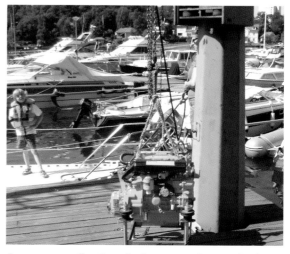

A crane on a floating dock was used to put in the new engine. It went very smoothly – in retrospect, I should have used this crane to remove the old engine.

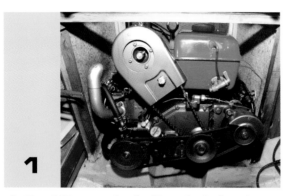

▲ The old Yanmar, that had been in the boat just over 30 years, had its own 5 litre fuel tank, and could be started with a crank. Now it was time for something new.

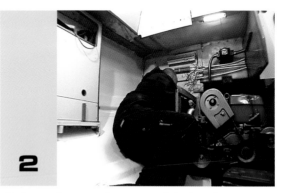

▲ I start by removing parts of the boat's interior to make enough room to get at the engine and work on it.

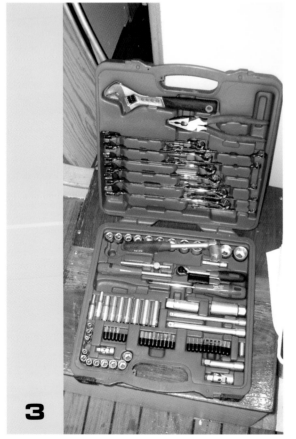

▲ A good quality set of socket wrenches made the job easier and was an excellent investment.

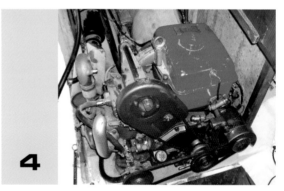

▲ In order to get the old engine out through the narrow companionwqy, I had to remove parts that made it too big, like the emptied integral diesal tank.

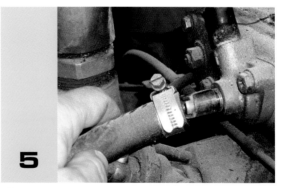

▲ The old engine was attached to the boat not only by the engine mounts but also by a cat's cradle of hoses, cables and wires.

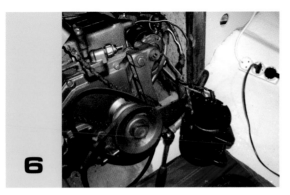

6

▲ The alternator was removed, and revealed a wiring system that had definitely seen better days. At some time in the past there had been a short circuit and some of the wiring insulation had melted.

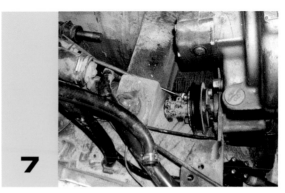

7

▲ The engine mounts and the shaft connection were removed last and the engine was ready to be lifted out.

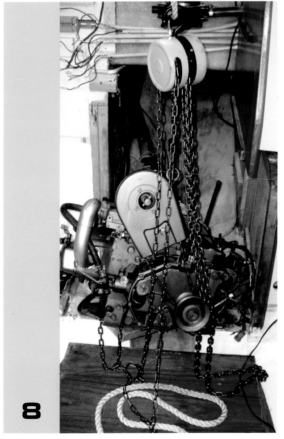

8

▲ When all the points of attachment had been disconnected, the engine could be raised by one person and in three steps be positioned on a piece of scrap plywood in the cabin.

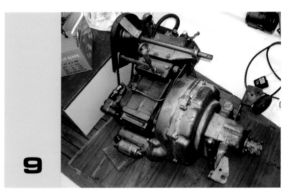

9

▲ The engine was left on protective plywood on the cabin sole for some time while I tried to work out how to get the engine out of the boat, now that it was high and dry in a tent for the winter project.

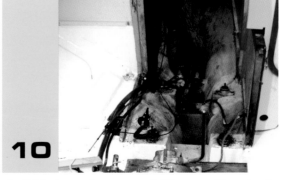

10

▲ With the engine removed, 30 years of ingrained dirt in the engine space became visible. Not an uplifting sight – it was like a dark hole.

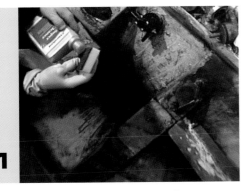

11

▲ Cleaning the bilge started with a high-pressure water wash and then continued with a scrub using a sponge, scouring pads and a degreasing agent.

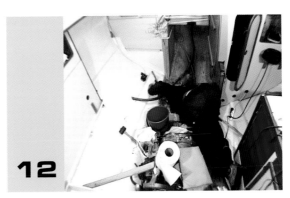

12

▲ It was awkward, cramped and difficult to reach the bottom of the bilge which was 80 cm/32 inches deep under the engine. But all loose paint and dirt had to be removed before I could paint.

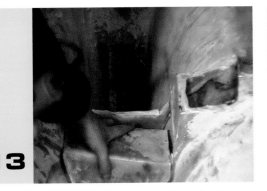

13

▲ At the same time I did some rough cutting for the new engine bed with the Fein oscillating saw (more about this in the next chapter).

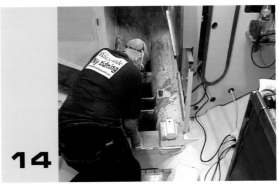

14

▲ After thorough cleaning, sanding and wiping with acetone, it was time to start painting with two-part paint.

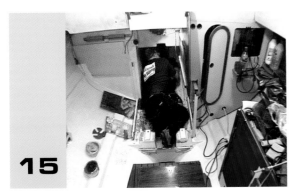

15

▲ On the wooden surfaces, I use alkyd paint so that these too would become easy to clean. However, a lot of this fine painting would end up behind the future fuel tank.

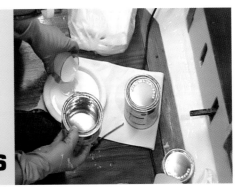

16

▲ Two-part paint must be correctly mixed in the right proportions. A proper measuring cup would have been better here but I used a plastic cup that I marked myself to make a perfectly sized batch for this job.

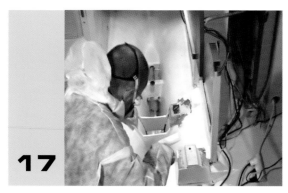

17

▲ Using a roller, I primed three times. I used a brush to get into hard-to-reach corners.

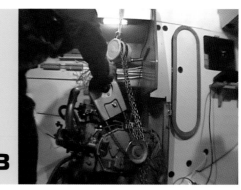

18

▲ I had taken off most of the removable parts but still had to roll the engine onto its side to get it out. With the chain hoist we prepared to lift the engine out of the cabin.

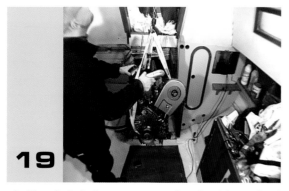

19

▲ The chain hoist was strapped to the ridge pole of the tent, which was supported by several temporary wooden posts. We tested the weight-carrying capacity of this arrangement and found it was adequate.

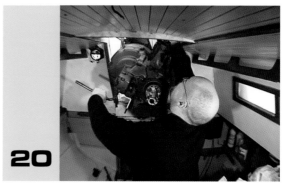

20

▲ To get the engine out of the compartment required a bit of maneuvering. We had to turn it onto its side to wriggle it out.

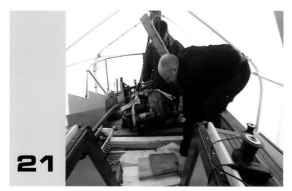

21

▲ Once it was in the cockpit we put the old engine down and moved the chain-hoist and support posts.

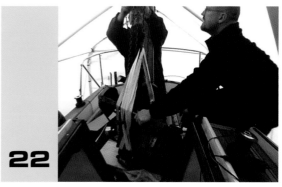

22

▲ We put the engine down every two feet to avoid overstressing the steel ridge pole.

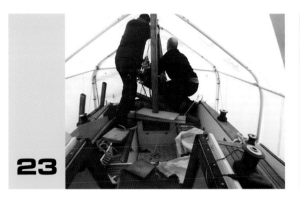

23

▲ In order to get the engine over the stern and down to the ground, we had to remove the stern rail, then install a long post behind the stern of the boat to support the ridge pole.

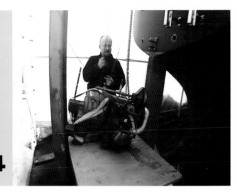

24

▲ The chain hoist did not reach all the way down to the ground, so we gave the engine a pit stop on a temporary wooden platform, while we lowered the chain hoist.

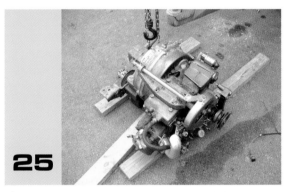

25

▲ The engine was finally on the ground, but it would have been easier to to this with the derrick on the dock.

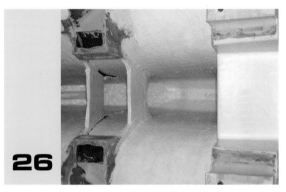

26

▲ Most of the engine space had been painted, except those areas that were going to need reworking in new fiberglass to make the new engine bed.

PROJECT LOG

LEVEL OF DIFFICULTY: easy

TIME SPENT: 5 hours to remove the engine + 10 hours for cleaning and painting

TOOLS AND EQUIPMENT USED: Socket wrenches, open-ended spanners, screw drivers, wire cutters, chain hoist, high pressure washer, rotary wire brush, angle grinder, fan.

MATERIALS CONSUMED: Two-part paint, brushes, rollers, roller pans, scouring pads, degreasing solution, acetone, rubber gloves, goggles, 'paper' suits.

03

THE NEW ENGINE BED

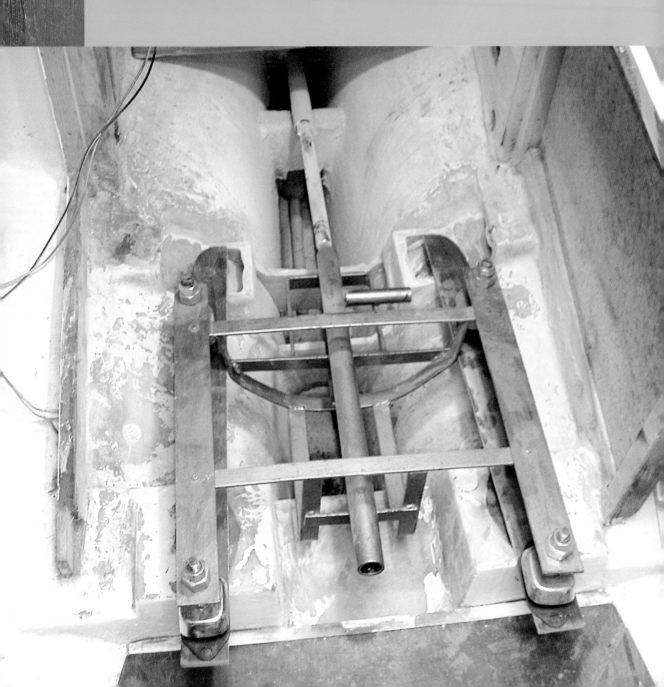

>> THE TRICKY ENGINE BED

When installing the new inboard engine, we had to modify the engine bed, which is something that requires great care and accuracy.

The size of the new engine can be critical if the engine space is small or obstructed by encroaching elements of other systems and the boat interior. As the project was just starting, I was still a bit worried about my ability to complete it by myself. However, I like a challenge and to learn new things, so with the promise of support from a skilled mechanic if I got stuck, I made a start.

If at all possible, I wanted to find an engine that wouldn't require any modification of the bed. But that didn't work out, and after getting advice from several skilled people, my worries were somewhat alleviated and I started modifying the engine space.

ADVICE FROM THE PROFESSIONALS

As my research proceeded, I realised that modifying the engine bed was not going to be simple. In fact there would be a lot of room for major error.

If the drive train includes a conventional one-piece prop shaft engine, a poorly aligned and dimensioned engine bed may make it impossible to complete the engine installation correctly. The engine and gearbox must be lined up, vertically and horizontally, with the propeller shaft in order to minimise vibration and abnormal wear. Confronting this requirement as a novice engine installer, I had to rework the engine bed without making any mistakes.

To increase my confidence before starting on this structural modification, I decided to ask Bo Linderholm from Ålstens Marine Tech to come and take a look at the boat.

Bo had promised to give me advice when I needed it. He'd been repowering boats for many years and gave me several tips on how I could complete my project efficiently and with a satisfactory result. Bo showed me where I needed to cut out existing structure and how to take measurements to get the new engine bed right.

Bo recommended that the new bed should be topped with flat steel bars, 10mm/ 3/8" thick, bolted through the new fibreglass onto the existing steel engine bearers or 'engine irons'.

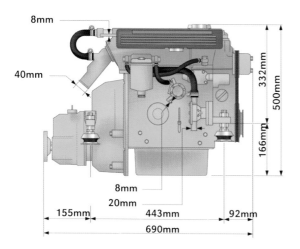

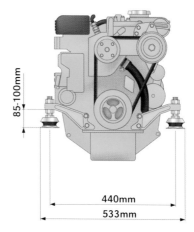

Make sure you check the measurements of the new engine, so it will fit into your available space. Often the most critical measurements are the distance between the mounts and how far below the engine the oil sump will reach. But also the total height and length of the new engine will

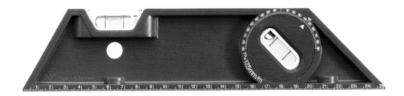

With the help of a spirit level or 'leaning level' with adjustable bubble (ie one in which the plastic tube with the bubble can be turned so that one sloping surface can be compared to, or made the same as, another sloping surface), I managed to get the new engine bed completely parallel with the shaft. The spirit level cost just under £15 at a large DIY store.

BEFORE STARTING

After having taken off all the old hoses, wires and cables, I lifted out the engine – a very awkward job in such a tight space. Once everything was out of the way, I measured the engine space and the spacing and length of the old engine irons. My new Vetus engine was almost exactly the same width as the old Yanmar, but was somewhat longer. The difference in length was manageable but the old Yanmar was assembled with engine attachments at different heights – something of a problem, which required lowering the aft support points of the engine bed.

Most engine-gearbox assemblies connected to a straight shaft must be tilted back so that the propeller shaft is angled down from the horizontal towards the stern. The angle at which the engine tilts back can be reduced with a down-angle gearbox. These are available from all marine gearbox manufacturers, and usually provide a down angle of 7° or 8°, allowing the engine to be closer to the horizontal; a desirable situation for internal lubrication.

An angled gearbox is standard on Volvo Penta's small engines, but for a small amount of money, all of the engines I considered could be supplied with a down angle gearbox. Of course, if you're getting a great deal on an engine, in my case buying a display model, you take the package 'as is'.

THE JIG

My expert contact lent me a jig for a couple of days. It made the job of sawing down the old engine bed considerably easier. I used a Fein oscillating electric saw for this hard work, which made it possible to saw straight into the existing fibreglass with very thin cuts.

The workspace was very cramped and a circular saw or reciprocating saw could not reach where I needed to cut. I cut the old steel engine irons with an angle grinder, keeping my face and body fully protected and keeping an extinguisher close at hand, just in case the shower of sparks and red hot steel started a fire – they didn't but better safe than sorry.

The best accessory to the jig was a spirit level with a bubble that could rotate to any angle. On *Roobarb* I got a shaft angle of 11° from the horizontal, which I transferred from the jig so that the long axes (plural of axis, not Viking weapons) of the new bearer irons were completely parallel with the shaft.

To get the irons flat steel bar on the same plane and level, I measured down from the top of the engine space and up from the hull, to the sidepieces of the jig, as I wasn't sure that the boat was completely level on the ground. Definitely a 'measure twice, cut once' situation.

I had to trust my own eyes when I centered the shaft in the shaft log, double checking with a carpenter's square set across the face of the stuffing box and other parts of the engine space that I thought should be square to the shaft. I made some wooden wedges to keep the old shaft correctly positioned, which in turn kept the jig on the right line for me to mark my cutting and filling lines. When I was close to completing the new engine bed a few days later, I once again borrowed the jig to double-check myself and put the finishing touches to the work.

CONSTRUCTION

After cutting off the unnecessary parts of the old engine bed, I cut two pieces of plywood to use as templates for the flat steel bars that would become the top of the rebuilt engine bed.

I remade these plywood templates several times, cutting and fitting to find the ideal shape and size that would get the real irons and the back of the engine as close to the hull as possible

With the help of these easily-adjustable plywood templates I could see that the front end of the engine needed to be raised by just over 20mm (¾"). I made shim plates from Forex Classic (a sheet product made of foamed polymer, left over from the fabrication of parts in the new interior), then formed the resulting slopes with high density, high strength epoxy filler. On *Roobarb* I was able to position the new engine 10–15cm (4" 6") further aft in the hull than the old one.

This meant that the new engine, although a bit longer, did not reach further forward in the cabin, which would have required rebuilding the companionway stairs, reducing the usable floor space. There was plenty of width in the engine compartment and the new diesel was going to be in the middle so it would have reasonable access all round.

Initially I had thought that it might be possible to make a storage rack within the engine space for maintenance parts such as filter elements, belts and impellers, but by the time the exhaust system, hoses,

filters, diesel tank, etc had been installed, I gave up on the storage rack idea – it was a tight space without adding optional extras.

TUNING

With the engine and its mounts temporarily in place (as an exact template), I marked the steel engine bearer irons and, after hoisting the engine out of the way, drilled holes in the irons and threaded them to receive 8mm stainless steel machine screws (ie bolts). I bought a simple threading tool with a lever (called a 'tap') for about £10.

The 10mm bolt holes in the engine mounts were a little larger than the machine screws, which gave me a couple of mm for adjustment should it be necessary before tightening the nuts (as it turned out to be).

For the front engine mounts I set things up so that an extra long bolt on each side could be screwed into the existing irons that were still in place below the new irons.

My expert contact also suggested having the new engine mounts one size larger than those normally delivered with the new engine. These mounts are actually intended for the slightly larger four cylinder engines supplied by Vetus, but they're working well on *Roobarb*.

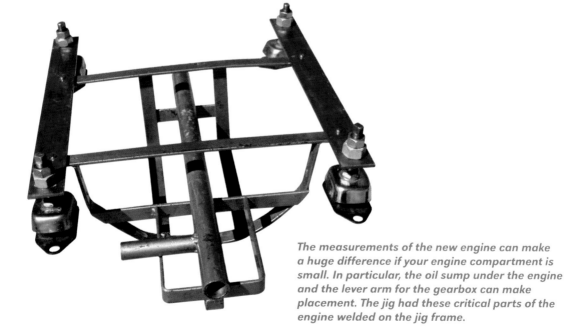

The measurements of the new engine can make a huge difference if your engine compartment is small. In particular, the oil sump under the engine and the lever arm for the gearbox can make placement. The jig had these critical parts of the engine welded on the jig frame.

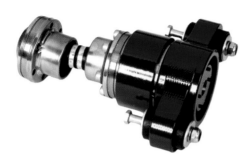

If your boat is equipped with a flexible coupling and thrust bearing assembly, with constant velocity joints, such as the devices supplied by Aquadrive, Python-Drive, Hydradrive and Vetus, the exact alignment of the shaft and engine/ gearbox assembly become less critical. These drive couplings can be very helpful to a do-it-yourself installer, if there's enough space to add one between the gearbox and prop shaft.

If your boat has a sail drive, it makes changing the engine much simpler as there are far fewer adjustments to be made to the engine bed.

ADDITIONAL ATTACHMENTS

Powerful forces are at work when a boat is rolling or pitching in big seas. Significant G-forces occur as the roll stops and reverses, as they do when the bow stops going down at the bottom of a trough or up at top of a wave. As the engine is one of the most heavy (more properly, massive) objects in the boat, these powerful G-forces put tremendous load, up and down, on the engine mounts and their connections to the engine bed.

THE FULL SCALE MODEL JIG

An acquaintance of mine replaced his thirty year old Yanmar YSE8 with a 16 hp inboard engine from Beta Marine. He bought a display engine at the end of an Autumn Boat Show. The way he made his jig was quite interesting.

The boat is a 1976 Compis 28 that has access to the engine room through a hatch in the cockpit floor and another way into the engine room from the galley. Since he selected an entirely new (then) engine model, there was no ready-to-use jig available, so he took the brochure drawings and with the help of the zoom function in a photocopier, extended them to create two full size installation drawings of the engine; one of the front and one of

the side. Using these expanded drawings, he made a model (a plywood model into which the engine would theoretically just fit). He used this full size model to find out if the engine could be manoeuvred down through the engine hatch and if it would be low enough to fit into the rather low compartment.

He remarked: 'It's really helpful to have a full-size lightweight model of the engine, especially when that engine has to be manoeuvred through narrow openings and into a tight space, tipping it this way and that to wriggle it through.

It's very difficult to figure out how to get an engine in, and if it will go in at all, just by measuring. You certainly don't want to use the real engine, weighing more than a hundred and twenty kilos (or 270 pounds) for these manoeuvring trials.'

The engine bed adaptor kit was provided by Sjoberg's Marine and Motor, a company with 30 years experience of selling and installing engines from Yanmar and Beta. The kit was made from flat bars of standard 'black iron' (mild steel) and then protected with anti-corrosion paint. He locked these new engine bearers firmly in place by bolting them down into the existing threaded holes in the old engine bed. The sequence opposite shows the whole process.

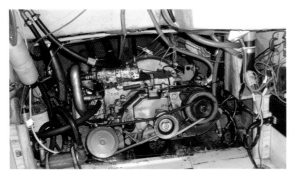

The old engine, a Yanmar YSE8, seen from the cabin side in an acquaintance's boat, a Compis 28.

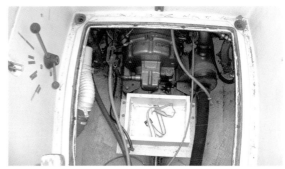

Looking down through the open hatch in the cockpit sole. This proved to be the easier of the two possible routes in for the new engine.

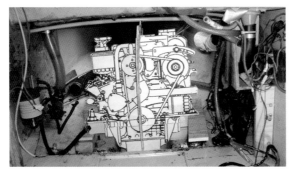

A full-scale model was made by using expanded drawings as templates for the plywood sides of the model. As an aid in visualizing the final installation and all the required connections, we then glued the drawings to the plywood.

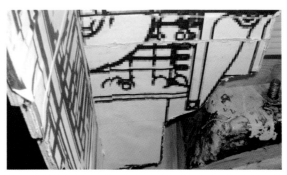

The oil sump under the engine is one of the critical measurements that has to be made to make sure there is enough space.

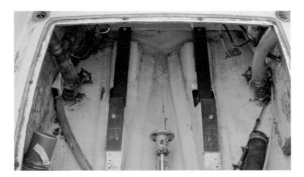

The engine bearer irons could be seen through the open hatch in the cockpit sole. We kept the old shaft, but added a flexible coupling. This would make the alignment process easier, to allow for irregularities in the shaft's rotation, and generally reduce vibration.

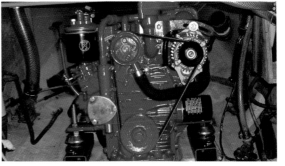

The engine was in place even though there were still things to attach. This photo was taken from the cabin, and you can see that all of the service points are easily accessible.

FOCUS ALTERNATIVE METHODS

Different boats require different approaches. The following are some good examples of both amateur and professional engine bed reconstruction. Most new engines fit surprisingly well onto old engine beds. New engines are considerably smaller than old engines of similar power output, but the manufacturers understand the installation issues and try to keep the mounts roughly the same size. That's why large-scale engine room reconstruction is not often required.

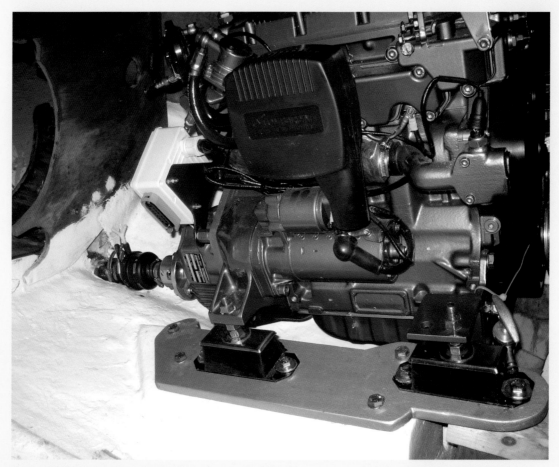

The old Yanmar YSB12 was replaced with a Lombardini 30 hp. model. You can see how the new bearer irons stick out about 10cm (3' 8") in front of the old engine bed and into the cabin. The engine was pushed into place over a slipway made of a wooden plank, as there was no room for a hoist under the cockpit, where the engine had to go. Sliding a diesel engine is difficult, and you've got to be very careful it doesn't topple over, damaging you, the boat and itself. 'Light' is a relative term when applied to engines – these machines are still very heavy compared with most things a novice installer has previously handled.

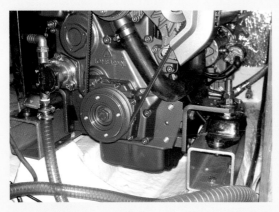

In a 37-footer the old Penta MD17 was replaced with a four cylinder, 60 hp Lombardini. In this case the engine attachments had to be given a substantial lift by bolting square section steel tubes to the engine bearers, bringing the new engine up to the required level.

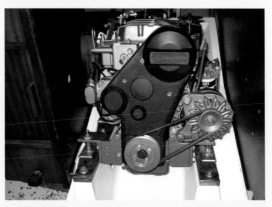

The owner of a 31-footer cut out new engine bearers from 16mm (5' 8") steel with an angle grinder. He cleaned, primed and painted the metal to resist corrosion and bolted the new bearers to the existing ones. The bolt holes in the new irons were elongated to allow for some sideways adjustment as the hold-down bolts were tightened.

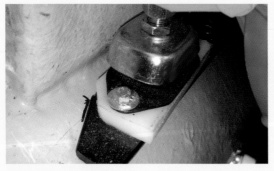

The captive bolts and double nuts on engine mounts provide for vertical adjustment, but if the captive bolt isn't long enough to get the engine into alignment, you may have to put some shim material under the mount to raise it.

There is a point at which a prudent installer is going to stop shimming and re-work the engine bed. A lot of that decision making will be depend on the width of the engine bearers – the bigger the shim plates and their seated area, the more stable they will be. Shims take the full weight of the engine, so the material you use has to be very strong and incompressible and the shim has to support the whole footprint of the mount. A pile of washers on the mounting bolts won't do it.

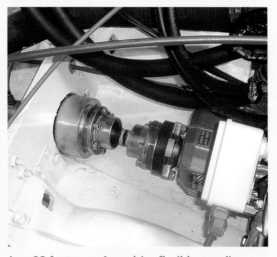

In a 29-footer an Aquadrive flexible coupling was installed, which has constant velocity joints and a thrust bearing to take the fore-and-aft forces from the propeller. More about constant velocity (cv) joints in Chapter 5.

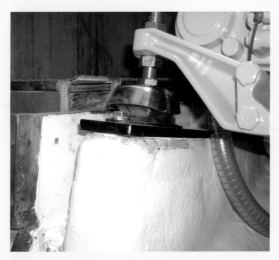

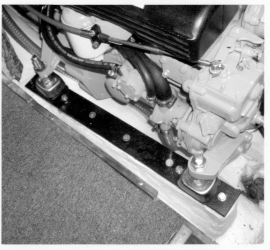

From the side of the bearer bars the countersunk bolt heads are flush and completely out of sight.

The new steel bearer bars are secured to the top of the existing engine bearers with countersunk bolts so that the heads of these bolts do not obstruct the new engine mounts. Five of these smaller bolts were used on each side to reduce the load on each one and spread the engine's weight across the engine bed and its bearers.

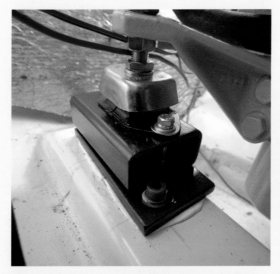

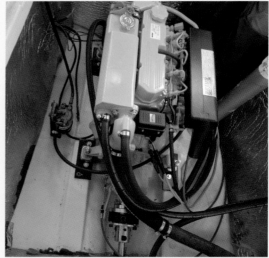

Here a section of steel tubing has been bolted down to a large, substantial and stable steel bearer plate. In this way you can often get the correct height without the need for fibreglass lamination work.

Same boat as left. For the back mounts flat steel was sufficient and it was possible to use the existing engine bed and bearer irons to support engine mounts at two levels without the need for extensive reconstruction.

>> STEP-BY-STEP

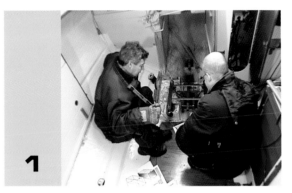

1

▲ The expert came to *Roobarb* and offered a lot of practical and useful advice on how to modify the engine bed.

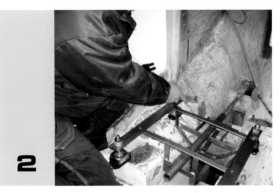

2

▲ With the help of the jig we were able to work out how the engine would fit and where we would need to cut and where we needed to build up with laminated fibreglass.

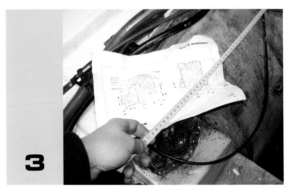

3

▲ I measured several times how the old engine bed needed to be cut to fit the new engine before I actually cut it.

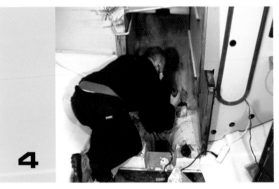

4

▲ The oscillating Fein saw did the job of cutting through the existing fibreglass around the old attachments fairly easily, even though it had to get through over 15mm (half an inch) of hard laminate.

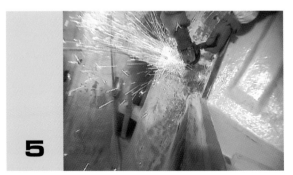

5

▲ The strong metal attachments of the old bearers at the back of the bed were cut away with an angle grinder.

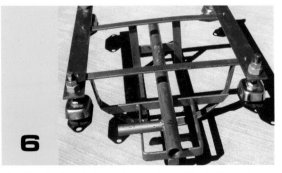

6

▲ The jig is fabricated with the critical dimensions of the oil sump, gearbox, engine legs, and the protruding shaft of the gear lever.

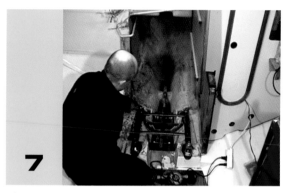

7

▲ The borrowed jig was used countless times to check my measurements and to check how the work with the new bed was progressing.

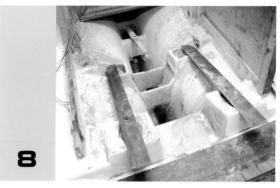

8

▲ I made prototypes engine bearer irons from plywood of the same size and thickness (10 mm or 3' 8") as the real irons.

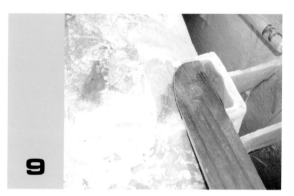

9

▲ At the rear attachment points the prototype templates showed where the top of the fibreglass bed needed to be ground down a bit.

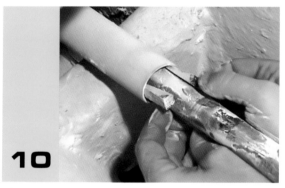

10

▲ Using small wooden wedges, I centered the old shaft exactly in the middle of the shaft log so that the shaft was held firmly in place while it carried and positioned the engine jig.

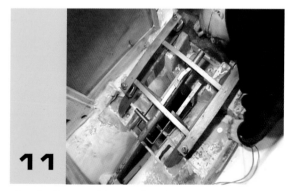

11

▲ The jig was slid onto the shaft and I sighted along it and the shaft tube of the jig to make sure that they were exactly lined up.

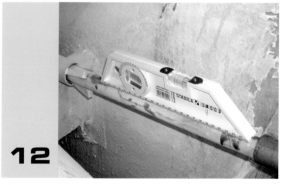

12

▲ I measured the down angle of the propeller shaft – on *Roobarb* it was 11 degrees.

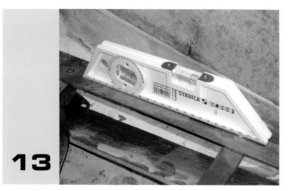

13

▲ The long axis of the jig must be parallel with the shaft. The adjustable level told me when it was at the same angle as the shaft and properly aligned.

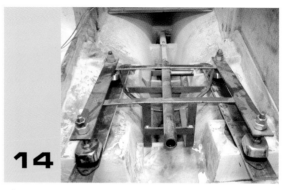

14

▲ The jig said that I had sawed and sanded away enough of the old engine bed. It also became apparent that the engine bed was too low at the front.

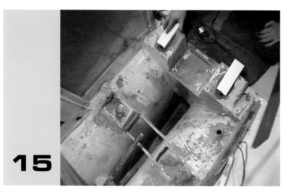

15

▲ To get the correct height at the front, I placed plastic pads of the required thickness under the front engine iron attachment points.

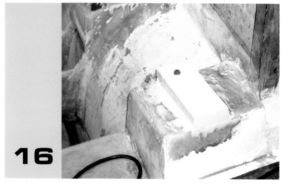

16

▲ I used a dense plastic material for these pads, epoxying them into place, and with recesses to allow later encasement in fibreglass.

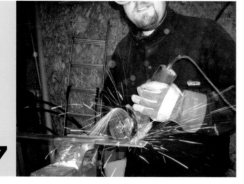

17

▲ I cut the steel engine bearer irons to the shapes developed on the plywood prototype templates.

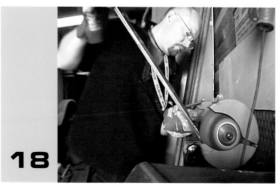

18

▲ The irons need to be bevelled to fit the shape of the hull. I made several 'cutting and fitting' trips to the boat to try the bearer irons in place in the engine room before I got them right.

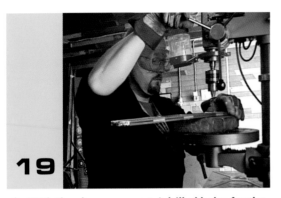

19

▲ With the shapes correct, I drilled holes for the bolts of the existing bed. They provided a very strong connection.

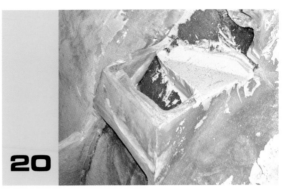

20

▲ Using the finalised irons as a guide, I could then create the support with epoxy resin. There wasn't much room for the rear attachments.

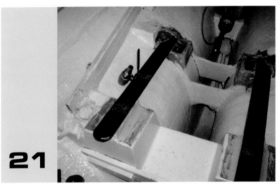

21

▲ The bearer irons are done and protrude five cm, in front of the old bed, although the weight of the new engine will still be centred above the old bed.

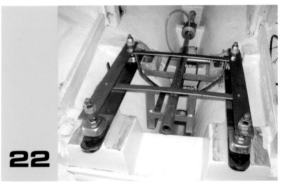

22

▲ Again, it's time to double check the alignment of the new engine bearers with the shaft, using the jig. The jig and the shaft align really well.

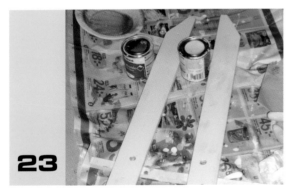

23

▲ The mild steel irons were cleaned, primed and painted with anti-corrosion paint.

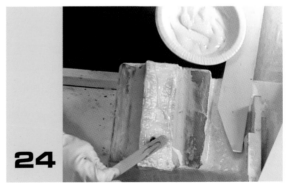

24

▲ The irons were bedded into thickened epoxy filler.

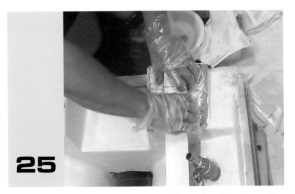

25

▲ The irons were then encased in a lamination of 3 layers of 300 gram chopped strand mat in epoxy resin.

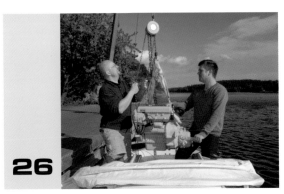

26

▲ With the boat back in the water, it was quite simple to lower in the new engine, using a dockside crane. Now it had to be installed.

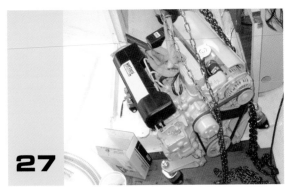

27

▲ Using the same thick wooden beam we used to get the old engine out, it proved relatively easy to move the new engine into place, in three steps – moving the beam back each time the engine was set down.

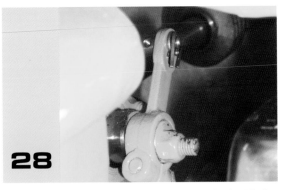

28

▲ All the critical dimensions were checked with the engine in place. The shaft of the gear shift lever just about fitted, but it was close.

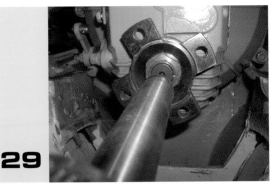

29

▲ The drive flange of the gearbox then needed to be aligned as exactly as possible with the new shaft.

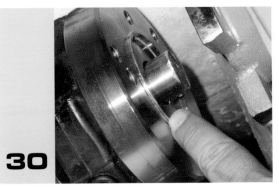

30

▲ The edge of the face plate of the flexible connection made it easy to see how well everything was lining up after adjustment. It was almost perfect.

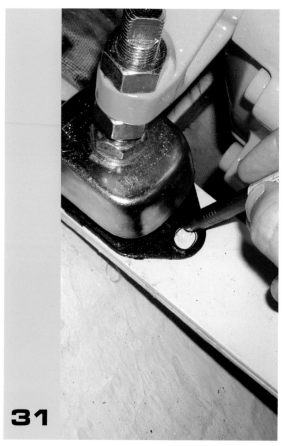

31

▲ To make receivers for the bolts for the new engine mounts, I marked the mounting hole locations then drilled down through the fibreglass to the new bearer irons.

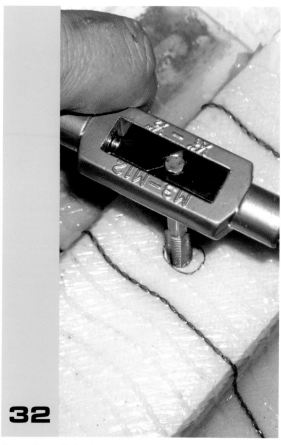

32

▲ I threaded all the holes with an 8mm tape. To be absolutely sure, I also put check nuts wherever I could.

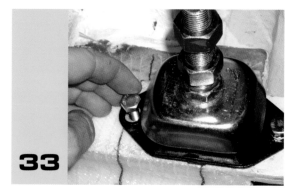

33

▲ In the bolt holes for the front engine mounts I had drilled all the way down to the steel of the sturdy original bearer irons and threaded those holes. With an extra long bolt, it made very strong attachments.

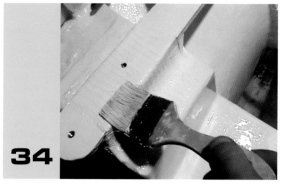

34

▲ All fibreglass surfaces received two coats of two part paint, so that they would be able to withstand oil and diesel drips.

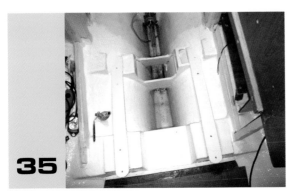

35

▲ The engine was now coming out one last time so that all the surrounding systems and accessories could be installed. The engine bed was tested and ready!

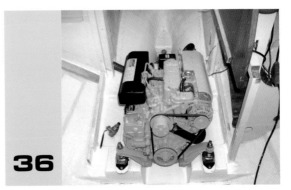

36

▲ I lowered the engine onto its new bed to see if everything had turned out the way I wanted. This was the second time the new engine had been tested for fit.

PROJECT LOG

LEVEL OF DIFFICULTY: difficult

TIME SPENT: 5 hours for measuring and double checking the measurements and then 20 hours for the construction work.

TOOLS AND EQUIPMENT USED: Owned or borrowed jig. Fibreglass laminating tools including shears, mixers, metal or polyethylene rollers, angle grinder. Respirator mask and goggles. Shop vac.

MATERIALS CONSUMED: Fibreglass combination matt/cloth, epoxy resin, hardener and filler, rubber gloves, resin application rollers, metal or plastic laminating rollers, chip brushes.

04

TANKS AND FUEL SYSTEMS

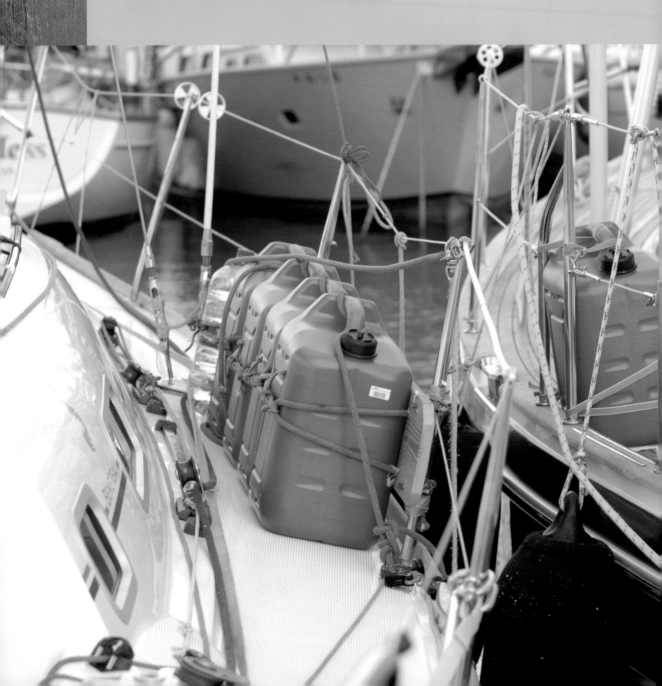

⟩⟩ FUEL FOR THOUGHTS

An old fuel system should be replaced when the engine is replaced, as there is a high probability of dried-out fuel hoses and the presence of decades of sediment and gunk at the bottom of the old tank.

Roobarb's 30 year old fuel system was replaced to meet stricter environmental standards, and to provide simple maintenance and long-distance cruising capability. And as it turned out, this part of the project wasn't all that simple.

The majority of fuel tanks on recreational boats are rarely, if ever, cleaned. One of the most common reasons for lifeboats being called out to boats is engine failure related to a blocked fuel system.

A common cause of such blockage is a filter clogged with dirt particles stirred up from the bottom of a badly contaminated fuel tank in rough conditions. The worse the weather, the more likely you are to get a problem. Running the tank near empty also causes the fuel system to suck in sediment and gunk from the bottom of the tank.

Another source of fuel system blockage is water in the diesel fuel. Micro-organisms can thrive in the boundary layer near the bottom of the tank, between the condensation water and diesel, becoming organic

muck that can clog filters and injector nozzles, the latter causing the engine to sputter constantly or even stop.

These problems have been made worse by the additives now mixed into diesel fuel (see fact box page 52).

I wanted to create a fuel system for the project boat *Roobarb* that would be easy to service and keep clean, especially as I hope to be soon sailing the seven seas.

I assumed that the engine would cut out sooner or later due to fuel problems – probably at the worst possible moment, so it must be easy to replace the filter and to bleed air from the fuel system.

MAIN TANK AND DAY TANK

The red metal fuel tank of the old Yanmar YSE12 was bolted directly to the engine. The previous owner, who built the boat, only used the engine occasionally and filled the tank with a hose from a jerry can.

My original idea for new fuel storage was to install a large main A4 stainless steel tank under the cockpit and a small tank with enough fuel for day

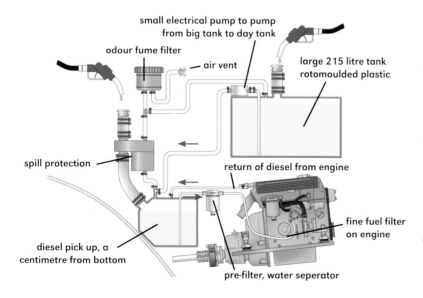

small electrical pump to pump from big tank to day tank

odour fume filter

air vent

large 215 litre tank rotomoulded plastic

spill protection

return of diesel from engine

diesel pick up, a centimetre from bottom

fine fuel filter on engine

pre-filter, water seperator

This illustration shows how Roobarb's system was finally set up. Fuel can be pumped from the main tank to the day tank when needed. But the 25 litre day tank also has its own filler cap. In an emergency, it's possible to connect the main tank directly to the engine, The 'splash-stop' takes care of possible spills while the day tank is being filled. The air vents from the main fuel tank and the day tank were joined, then connected to the fuel filter. Earthing/grounding cables are not shown in this sketch

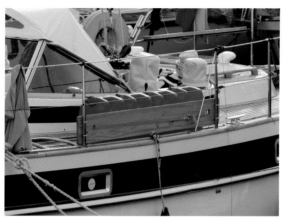

A Hallberg Rassy, the day before crossing the Atlantic with the ARC, with 100 litres of extra diesel secured to a board bolted to the lifeline stanchions.

sailing and short cruises. This small day tank would be positioned above the engine and hence feed by gravity if there would be a problem with the fuel pump on the engine.

The first plan for the main tank was to divide it in two tanks side-by-side, so that the free surfaces of liquid would be smaller. A high narrow tank is easier to draw fuel from because the level of the fuel in the tank does not change much when the boat heels. If the tank is wide and the fuel is able to splash and surge around, the fuel pipe may start sucking air, resulting in an engine shutdown in the thick of dealing with rough conditions.

After some modification, I stuck with these first ideas. I could see several advantages in filling the main tank with a lot of fuel for long distance ocean cruising (perhaps filling up in places where diesel is less expensive). And when sailing along the coast I would use the smaller day tank only, where you're always close to a fuel dock. The smaller tank would be the main source for fuel, and when empty at sea I would transfer from the big tank.

If my plan had been to go summer sailing only in European waters, the smaller tank would have been quite adequate on its own – there aren't many motoring hours between operational fuel docks in the sunny season. Another advantage of having a large permanent tank for long-distance cruising is that you don't need to have extra fuel in portable tanks on deck. On-deck tanks get in the way and reduce the stability

of the boat by moving its centre of gravity upwards. Several hundred extra kilos/pounds on deck make it more difficult for the boat to right itself, although even a large permanent tank below deck is still likely to have its centre of gravity above the water line.

The material in the tanks was first to be in stainless steel, but the size and weight made it an awkward solution, instead I opted for rotation moulded linear polythene.

ACCESSIBILITY

I also wanted a way to drain out condensed water, which is heavier than diesel and collects at the bottom of the tank.

A V-shaped tank with a sump (small collector pocket at the bottom) and drain valve would have been a simple solution, but I was persuaded not to do this by several people who said that sooner or later such a valve would break, allowing diesel fuel to empty into the bilge – a very unpleasant and potentially disastrous situation. According to CE rules it is permitted to have this solution for diesel, but not for petrol. I wanted to be on the safe side and chose not to pursue this idea.

A better approach is to permanently tilt the tank a few degrees, to create a low point from which you can suck out water and dirt with a hose and pump, inserted through an inspection or fill port in the top of the tank. This also allows you to remove algae and bacteria living in the boundary layer between water

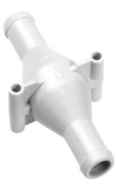

Another type of level control, The Fuel Whistle lets you hear when the tank is full. The Fuel Whistle is inserted in the vent line of the tank and whistles for as long as fuel is displacing the air in the tank. The whistling stops when the fuel reaches The Fuel Whistle, telling you to stop pumping – the tank is full.

and diesel, near the bottom of the tank. Cleaning out a diesel tank is not a fun job but it's got to be done on a regular schedule – I have learned the hard way. Working through the inspection port, you can suck up dirt and water from the bottom of the tank with a pump and a hose – a 6 litre/1.5 gallon vacuum-operated oil-changing pump is a low cost solution for a suitable pump. I made the small day tank detachable so that I could bring it ashore to give it a thorough cleaning, whenever necessary.

REFUELLING

The location of the re-fuelling fittings (deck fills) also required some thought. The decision to have two tanks meant that the plan of having one single opening for fuelling had to be abandoned.

The location of deck fills should be given careful attention – far too often they are found near the cockpit, at the lowest point on the deck and susceptible to water infiltration, which is a serious problem. There also needs to be a full-tank warning or control device so that diesel cannot overflow through the vent pipe into the water. Strict laws governing this have been enacted in many countries and are likely to be adopted worldwide.

As I wanted to make an environmentally responsible installation from the start, I elected to install a spill prevention device under the fill fitting of the day tank. The alternative was to use some other type of protection that would prevent diesel from escaping into the water, such as a catch filter on the bilge pump discharge – the main route overboard for fuel and oil spilled inside the boat.

The first idea was to weld a tank in stainless steel, but it turned out to be simpler and cheaper to fit a standard tank, and Vetus also had them on the shelf which speeded up my project.

To be able to fill the large tank, I needed to rebuild the Vetus connecting kit so it could be filled from the top. The solution was to re-weld and shorten the sleeve coupling, so that it fitted straight onto the connection kit. I asked a welder to help me with this job.

My plan was that before starting to fill up with diesel, I would use a small funnel with a built-in Teflon-covered stainless steel filter (known as a 'Baja filter' in the US). This filter prevented bigger dirt

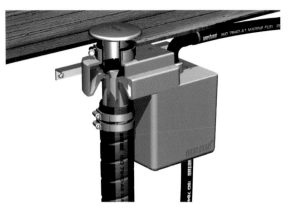

The 'splash-stop' takes care of possible spills while the day tank is being filled. The air vents from the main fuel tank and the day tank were joined, then connected to a fume filter.

particles and water from the filling stations storage tanks getting into the boat tanks, which is not uncommon in many places – even at one's home port.

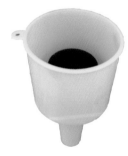

The funnel had the disadvantage of considerably slowing the fill rate, and quite often was only used at dodgy looking stations. It was also too small – I should have bought a bigger model that didn't overflow that easily. I sometimes followed the practice of some experienced long distance sailors, and used a filter funnel for the first ten litres of fuel, and if inspection then showed no dirt or water in the filter media, completed fuelling without the filter.

FUEL GAUGE

With any tank there should be a method of measuring the fuel level. To run out of fuel with a diesel engine is a pain in the neck, as the fuel system on the engine will probably need to be bled to get all the air out before you can start the engine again. There are

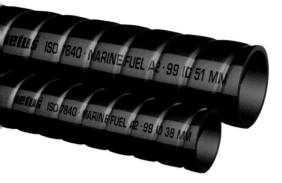

Buy good quality hose to connect the deck fill to the tank. The standard sizes are 51 and 38mm. This hose is expensive so measure twice before you buy it.

many different tank gauges on the market, both mechanical (with a float) and electronic (with a static sensor or ultrasound). If the fuel fill is directly above the tank, with a straight hose connection, that allows a rigid probe to reach the lowest point of the tank. The simplest way to check the tank is to use a graded dipstick, and this method worked well for the big tank on *Roobarb*.

The first time the tank was filled with diesel, I was there to make a notch on the dipstick for every 20 litres of fuel I put in. That dipstick is now stowed away from dirt and dust in a box right next to the fuel fill. The fuel fill hose on the day tank was curved, so a dipstick would not work as it did on the main tank.

Both tanks are made out of white, translucent plastic and in the right light it's possible to see the fuel level. The day tank is located in the bottom of a storage bin, and for a while I thought about making a glazed opening between the cabin and the tank space to provide a view of the fuel level in the tank from the cabin.

In the future I may add a small gauge to the day tank, as I now have to crawl into the cockpit storage compartment to visually check the level in the tank. It's not difficult but it is annoying to do when there's a lot of swell or it's raining heavily.

REGULATIONS

In a used recreational boat not many rules apply apart from the requirement that the tank should be properly fastened on board applies. Some countries have their own laws and regulations (ABYC in USA, for example) for fuel tanks, but if you are buying a tank from a reputable marine equipment dealer you can be reasonably sure that it will be in compliance with those laws and regulations, providing that you install the new tank in accordance with the manufacturer's recommendations. The rules and regulations applying to boat manufacturers are quite strict – you can read more about CE-regulations in a fact box in this chapter.

EARTHING/GROUNDING

When fuel flows it creates static electricity, with a potential difference that can be as high as ten thousand volts. The possibility of a spark from this static electricity is a significant fire hazard.

With that in mind, all metal parts of a marine fuel system must be earthed/grounded with a multi-strand bonding cable. These cables need to connect the deck fill, tank, metal pipes, valves, filters etc to the earthing/grounding point on the engine or better, to an earth/ground plate in the hull hopefully if the boat has one, if not one can be fitted.

The metal nozzle of the fuel dock pump hose also needs to be earthed/grounded by keeping it touched to the metal edge of the boat's deck fill fitting throughout the fuelling process.

With a plastic tank, things are not so clear cut, but the deck fill is nearly always made of metal, and needs to be earthed/grounded regardless of the tank material. The experts didn't give me consistent opinions on this subject and I'm going to look for ways to improve the earthing/ grounding on *Roobarb*'s fuel system.

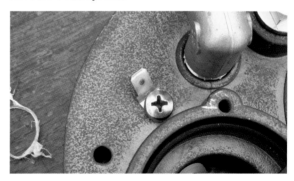

On this metal tank top, where all fuel hoses are connected, there's an earthing/grounding screw that must be bonded to the boat's earth/ground and to the other metal parts of the fuel system.

HOSES

Something that's easy to overlook when you're putting together the budget for an engine replacement is the cost of the many metres of hose of various types that you're going to need. High quality marine hoses are expensive, for example, the exhaust hose for *Roobarb*'s new engine has a list price of more than £25/$40 per metre, without VAT/ sales tax. 8 mm marine grade fuel hose (between the tank and the engine) costs about £6/$10 per metre, while 51 mm fuel fill hose (between the deck fill and the tank) costs about £40/$64 per metre. It's a good idea to take careful hose measurements before you visit the chandler – this is expensive stuff, and if it's too short, no matter how many times you cut it, will still be too short.

FUEL FILTER

I installed a pre-filter between the tank and the engine to protect and supplement the fine filter mounted on the engine between the fuel lift pump and the high-pressure injection pump. This filter on the engine is not intended to be the only fuel filter, there must be a good quality pre-filter to separate out water and dirt particles, so that the filter on the engine works as a last resort and only has to catch the very last, fine fuel contaminants that get through the pre-filter. (More about filters in Chapter 6.)

MICRO-ORGANISMS

Micro-organisms can be found in the boundary layer between water and diesel, and they feed on the carbon in the diesel fuel. This can cause clogging of

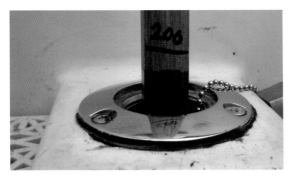

It's necessary to have a way of measuring the fuel level in the tanks. This can be a dipstick or an electric/electronic fuel gauge.

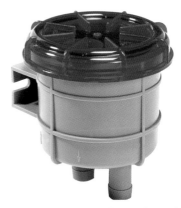

This device prevents diesel fumes from drifting into the cockpit from the overboard vent. Many countries require a fuel spill prevention device – a regulation that is certain to apply everywhere in the near future. On Roobarb, I installed a Vetus 'Splash-Stop' under the fill fitting of the day tank.

the filter, uneven fuel consumption and a sputtering or stopped engine.

Especially in the winter, condensation occurs in the fuel tank of the boat, and creates the water necessary for microbe growth. SPI does not recommend adding a fuel conditioning agent containing biocides to stored diesel.

Dead microbes form an organic gel (gunk) that clogs the fuel filters and injection nozzles, causing the engine to run rough or stop. SPI say that the only environmentally-friendly way of stopping the multiplication of the microbes is to remove their habitat. This is done by reducing the risk of water getting into fuel tank by keeping the tank full of fuel to minimize the intrusion of moist air from the vent pipe. It's also important to regularly remove water from the tank.

The amount of FAME/bio-diesel blended into boat diesel varies from company to company. You can try asking the staff at the fuel dock about the content of their fuel, but they probably won't know. To get the facts you'd have to trace the delivered fuel back to the refinery.

More info: The British Marine Federation's website (www.britishmarine.co.uk) has some interesting articles, as does the US Environmental Protection Agency's site (www.epa.gov), and these can be down loaded by anyone wanting to learn more about the use of bio-diesel in boats.

FOCUS | LOW SULPHUR DIESEL

For several years now, environmentally-friendly, low sulphur diesel has been readily available at fuel docks (environmental class 1 diesel is free of sulphur, with a low aromatic hydrocarbon content).

However, depending on where you sail, diesel fuel may contain a small amount of fatty acid methylene ester (FAME), aka bio-diesel, without it being listed or shown at the pump, and some boaters add as much as 25% bio-diesel to their mineral oil based diesel fuel, as an environmentally beneficial action.

Unfortunately, there are some unintended consequences of using fuel mixtures containing bio-diesel, including the possibility of accelerated deterioration of seal materials and hoses, and – more significantly for most boaters – an increase in the growth of micro-organisms at the fuel-water boundary layer in the tank plus the accumulation of gunk at the bottom of the tank.

To minimize this increase in biological activity and its damaging consequences for a boat's fuel system, fuel containing bio-diesel (FAME if you prefer) should not be left in the fuel tank for prolonged periods, such as over the winter.

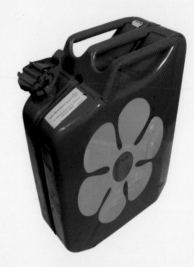

Some countries have regulations also limiting the storage time for these fuels on land. This is particularly applicable to recreational boats, which often sit for long periods of time without use, with partially full tanks. Using the small tank on *Roobarb* for day sailing and short trips should protect the fuel system, as the fuel in that tank will be used and replaced frequently.

FOCUS | CLEANING FUEL TANKS

If there is reason to believe that there are micro-organisms and gunk in the tank, it will have to be cleaned by hand. Powerful biocides (chemicals that kill algae and micro-organisms) are available but opinions vary as to whether they should be used. Even if the microbes die, they don't disappear but instead sink to the bottom of the tank as an organic gel (gunk) and may clog your filters the next time the sea gets rough enough to stir up the contents of the fuel tank.

To mechanically clean a tank, you first empty it of diesel fuel, which can be stored for re-use if it is completely clean and clear. If you have any doubts about its condition, take the old fuel to the recycling centre. If you're lucky, the tank will have an inspection port through which you can insert the wand of a steam cleaner or a stick wrapped in absorbent cloth. If the tank has a low point or a sump, it's best to start by cleaning there. If access is cramped, or the tank has an irregular shape, you may have to make some special tools, to reach all the nooks and crannies.

SOME TIPS ABOUT HANDLING FUEL

- The risk of condensation forming in the fuel tank is reduced if the tank is full, with little or no airspace above the diesel fuel. This is especially important for long lay-ups including winter storage.
- Either fill or empty the tank if possible. Emptying it is recommended if you use environmental diesel.
- Fill up at fuel docks that sell a lot of diesel, where you have enjoyed good service in the past. If that's not possible, pump the diesel into a fuel can, then pour from the can into the tank through a funnel with a water separating filter element.
- Drain the water out of the tank every year. Some tanks can be emptied through a bottom drain. Similarly, drain the water from the canister of the fuel/water separator filter frequently, so that that water never gets pumped into the engine.
- Do not use additives that claim to remove water from fuel – the laws of physics and chemistry have not been suspended, even for recreational boats. These additives usually contain alcohol of one sort or another, and absorb or suspend

water. The resulting liquid flows unimpeded through your fuel water separator filter and reaches your engine injectors and cylinders, where the water part of it turns into steam. This is not good as it puts unpredictable stresses on the internal parts of your engine. Let's leave these products to people who wish to run steam engines on diesel.

- Make sure that your deck fill and vent line breather fitting are installed in places where they won't let water drip or pour into the tank. If the deck fill is under a puddle, mop it up before you open the fill.
- Install a water separating filter of high quality as a complement to the engine's fine filter.
- Don't penny-pinch and don't underestimate! Think about the replacement cost of the engine you are protecting!
- Add a high water alarm to the water bowl of your fuel/water separator filter.
- Remember that common rail diesel engines, with very high injection pressures, are even more susceptible to damage from contaminated fuel than conventionally injected engines. Lack of attention to routine maintenance and carelessness when selecting and changing filter elements can have very expensive consequences.

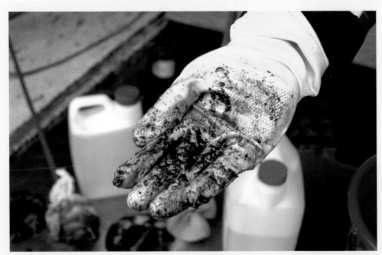

It's essential to clean a diesel tank from time to time. There can be many particles at the bottom, in the worst case 'diesel critters' – living micro organisms including algae.

FOCUS ORDERING A STAINLESS STEEL TANK

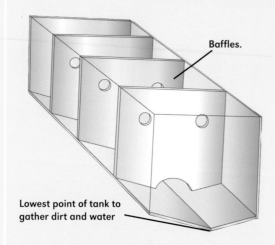

Baffles.

Lowest point of tank to gather dirt and water

This is a preliminary sketch of the main tank, fabricated in stainless steel, that would fit under the cockpit. The triangular underside that would follow the shape of the hull and create a low point where dirt and water could collect and be removed. I received a couple of quotes on the large stainless tank, both around £1100/$800. The empty tank would weigh about 65 kilo/143 pounds.

When I thought about the cost and then the difficulty of getting that big, heavy tank through the companionway hatch, I went with a less expensive, smaller and much lighter roto-molded polyethylene tank instead.

The welder said that when he gets a tank order, there are several factors that decide how the end product will look. A tank has to be designed, sized and fabricated to suit the boating activities of the customer, in particular how long he wants to be able to motor between refuelling stops.

The space available also plays a big role in designing the tank. The welder went on to say that he needs at least a drawing of the new tank from the customer, but a full-scale model made of cardboard, masonite or thin plywood is much better, because the boat owner has been able to check his ideas for installation and fit. Per also said that the customer needs to indicate where he or she want to position all of the hose connections – fill, supply, return and ventilation/breathe and the inspection port if required.

If you are going to have an inspection port (and you should) to facilitate cleaning the tank, you need to be sure that it is placed where there's enough room for you to work over it.

The type of stainless steel selected depends on the size of the tank and in what way the boat is going to be used. 1.25 mm stainless steel

is normally specified (rust-resistant SIS 2333/BS3605-G801/ASTM A312-TP304/18/8) which is not acid resistant.

However a fast motor boat may need stronger tanks to withstand the loads created as it pounds through big seas. In those cases it may be appropriate to go up to 1.5 or 2 mm stainless.

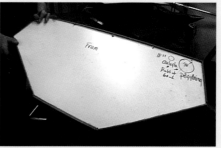

A boat owner has given the welder a full size hardboard model for a new tank. All the connections have been drawn on the model in their required locations, and the model has been tested for passage through the companionway hatch and for fit under the cabin sole, in the bilge.

FOCUS CE-RULES FOR PERMANENTLY INSTALLED DIESEL TANKS

MATERIAL MINIMUM THICKNESSES FOR STRENGTH AND CORROSION RESISTANCE

Aluminium alloy (may not contain more than 0.1% copper)	2.0 mm
Stainless steel	1.0 mm
Mild steel plate	2.0 mm
Hot dipped galvanized steel plate	1.5 mm

The standards ISO 21487 & 16147 define what materials may be used for manufacturing diesel tanks and how these tanks should be constructed and tested. The rules cover new boats but provide good guidelines for fabricating and fitting a tank into an existing boat.

All materials used in the fuel system must to be resistant to all of the chemicals to which the system will normally be exposed. These include grease, oil, fuel, cleaning agents and salt water.

The melting point of plastic fuel system components must be above 150°C. Copper pipes may be used for all connections, but must be galvanically separated from mild steel, aluminum and zinc plated (galvanized) steel used in tanks and other metal fuel system components.

Tanks of all materials must withstand a pressure test for leakage. Plastic tanks must also be tested for fire resistance.

If a tank is equipped with baffles, their cross-sections must not take up more than 30% of the total cross section of the long axis of the tank. The limber holes in the baffles must be shaped and positioned so that the fuel can drain along the bottom of the tank to the suction pipe and the baffles must also not allow fuel vapour to be trapped in any upper part of the tank, away from the ventilation/breather fitting.

The filling pipe/hose of the tank must have an inner diameter of at least 31.5 mm. Ventilation/breather connections to the tank must have an inner diameter of atleast 11 mm.

The tank must be attached to the hull in such a way that if the tank breaks loose, the integrity of the hull is not impaired. The installation materials used to attach the tank to hull should be strong enough for the application and formed of corrosion resistant metal or fabric. It must be possible to determine the level in a tank.

The ISO rules describe in a few words how a tank should be designed and what requirements the authorities impose on boat builders when it comes to installing tanks.

>> STEP-BY-STEP

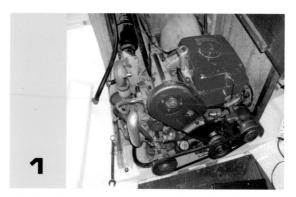

1

▲ The old engine had a small day tank of five litres that was bolted directly to the engine. It was filled from a jerry can about every five running hours.

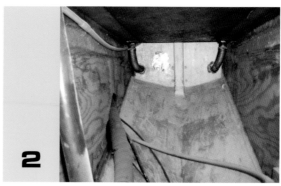

2

▲ When the engine had been taken out, I could get access to the space under the cockpit. This void had before acted as an effective amplifier of the engine noise.

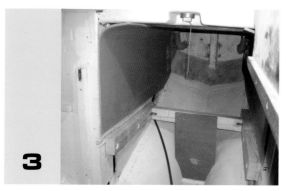

3

▲ The first step after painting the space was to make a sturdy platform that would hold a full tank (approx 180 kilos/396 pounds).

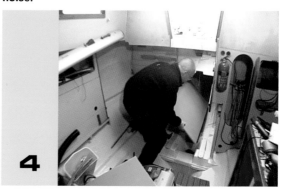

4

▲ All touching surfaces were padded with foam plastic to prevent chafing. The tank fitted with only a couple of centimetres to spare.

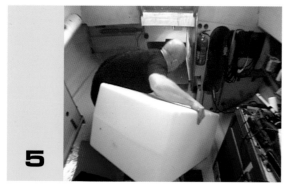

5

▲ After deciding not to go with a stainless steel tank, I tested that a standard plastic tank could be used.

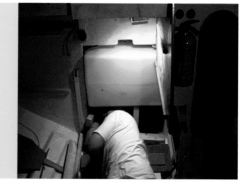

6

▲ After some manoeuvring, I managed to position the roto-moulded polyethylene tank, with a 215 litre capacity in the space under the cockpit.

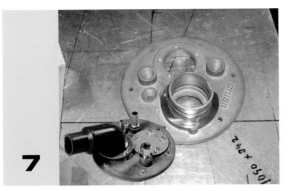

7 ▲ The fill connector fitting had to be cut in two. One part of the pipe was welded onto the base flange of the connection kit.

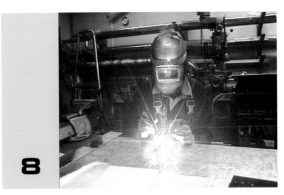

8 ▲ An elbow was needed to fit the breather hose to the tank vent. Several layers of plumber's Teflon tape ensured that the seals were good.

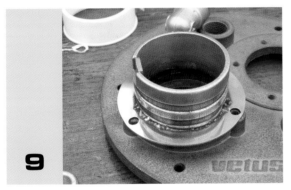

9 ▲ The welding made it possible to fill from straight above the tank rather than from the side as in the original kit.

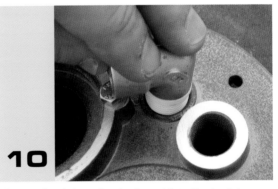

10 ▲ An aluminium ring is slotted into the tank to form a backing collar, with threaded receiver holes for the screws securing the base flange of the connection kit. A large 'o'-ring prevented leakage through the slots.

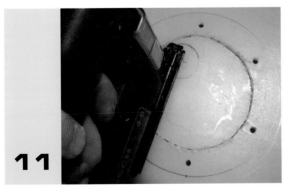

11 ▲ An opening was cut in the big tank for the connection kit. The tank deflated somewhat when I drilled the first hole and it became significantly smaller.

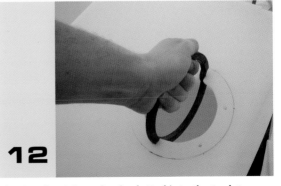

12 ▲ An aluminium ring is slotted into the tank to form a backing collar. A large 'o'-ring prevented leakage through the slots.

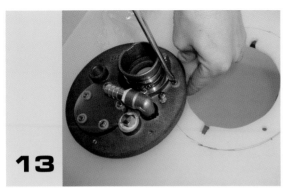

13

▲ After some manoeuvring, I managed to position a roto-moulded polyethylene tank, with a 215 litre capacity. It turned out to be very close to a perfect fit.

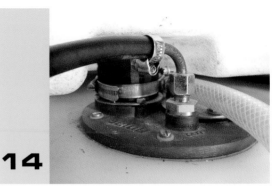

14

▲ There was a recess in the underside cockpit where I got the connection kit to fit with some difficulty. A short length of fuel fill hose, pre-installed on the connection kit, made hooking things up a bit easier.

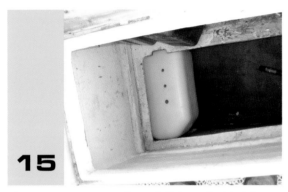

15

▲ After trying several possibilities, I decided that the best location for the day tank would be in the storage locker on the starboard side of the cockpit.

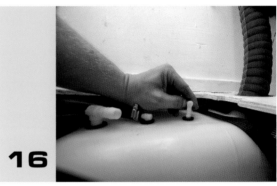

16

▲ The small day tank was secured with straps so that it could be taken out and cleaned from time to time. The fuel, return and vent hose goes on the top.

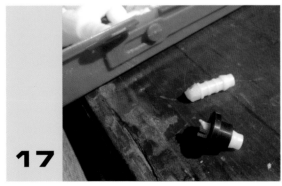

17

▲ The 8 mm connections to the day tank were made of plastic and two of them broke – they weren't strong enough for this application. Eventually, I found replacements at the local hardware store.

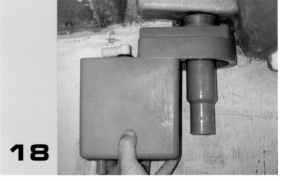

18

▲ There was just about enough room for the 'Splash-Stop' spill control device under the deck fill in the storage locker. It was a tight fit and I had to cut a bulkhead to get it in.

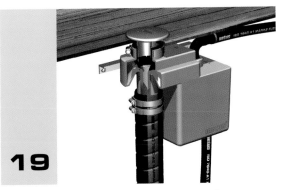

19

▲ The 'Splash-Stop' prevents diesel fuel from foaming up the fill hose and spilling into the water. Now there is a smaller version with same funtion.

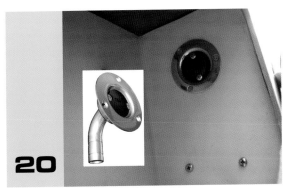

20

▲ I placed the fuel tank breather skin fitting in a well protected spot in a cockpit locket. I had added a 'no-smell' filter in the vent line to stop diesel fumes getting into the cockpit.

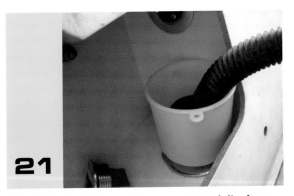

21

▲ A filter in this funnel stops water and dirt from reaching the tank. Unfortunately, it takes a long time to fill the tank through this very useful device.

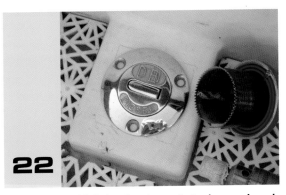

22

▲ The deck fill fitting for the main tank was placed in the floor of the cockpit, on a raised pad to protect it from standing water.

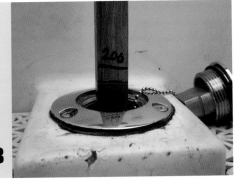

23

▲ The fuel level in the main tank can be measured with a graduated dipstick, inserted down into the tank through the deck fill.

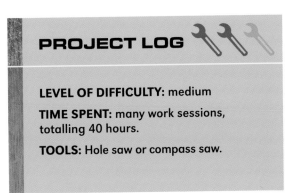

PROJECT LOG

LEVEL OF DIFFICULTY: medium

TIME SPENT: many work sessions, totalling 40 hours.

TOOLS: Hole saw or compass saw.

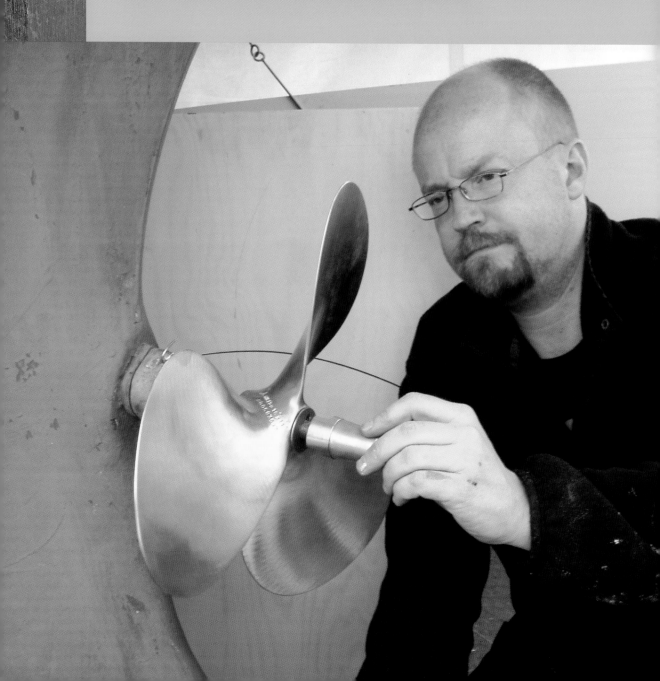

05
PROPELLERS AND STERN GEAR

>> PROPULSION

To select a propeller, you need to take several issues into account. And it can get a bit theoretical, so bear with me. In the end you will probably just take the advice from the propeller expert that sells you the propeller.

The drive train consists of the engine and its mounts, the gearbox and the running or stern gear (shaft, shaft couplings, shaft bearings, seals, struts and the propeller). Selecting the right propeller for a particular boat is quite a complicated task, but if you seek the assistance of a reputable and well-established propeller shop, the knowledge and experience of the sales people and technicians will take most of the guesswork out of the selection process.

There are charts (nomograms) available that can be used to identify the correct propeller configuration (diameter, pitch, number and size of blades etc.) but the input of an experienced propeller salesman is going to be the most important and reliable information available to the first-time engine installer.

A propeller is described by its diameter, pitch, number of blades, area of one blade and the direction of rotation. Today there are computer programs that calculate and describe each of these elements of a propeller, and free downloads are available on the net for those who'd like to try it themselves.

Changing the shaft and propeller at the same time is relatively painless – they will be ordered to fit each other, but if you want to use an existing shaft to turn a new prop, there may be some problems to overcome. There has always been a variety of prop to shaft connections (Volvo Penta, for example, have had their own propeller shafts with non-standard keyways and unusual thread gauges), but now there are innumerable variations of attachment details, and without great care and accuracy in matching a new prop to an existing shaft, you may end up being stuck with a prop that doesn't fit, and perhaps having to search for a used prop that will fit. You can't go far wrong by taking the existing shaft to the prop shop at the beginning of the buying process.

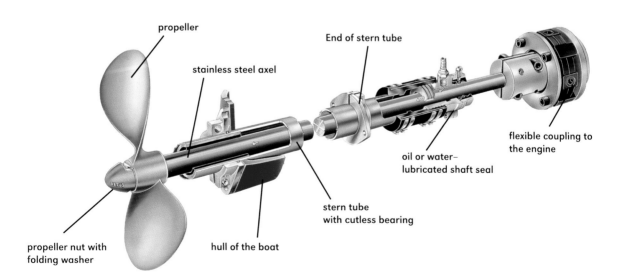

propeller

stainless steel axel

End of stern tube

flexible coupling to the engine

oil or water–lubricated shaft seal

stern tube with cutless bearing

propeller nut with folding washer

hull of the boat

Cross section of the drive train on a sailing yacht.

UNDERSTANDING PROP ROTATION

The diameter of a propeller is the diameter of the circle described by a 360° rotation of the outermost points of the blade tips. The pitch of a propeller is the theoretical distance that it would move along the axis of the propeller shaft if rotated 360° in a solid medium. A good way to visualize this is to observe how much a nut moves along a bolt when the nut is turned through one full rotation. It's not a perfect analogy, though, because propeller blades function more like wings than screw threads, with a pressure difference between one side of the blade and the other side, resulting in lift or propelling force.

The direction of rotation, left hand or right hand, also forms a part of the specification of a propeller. To determine the direction of rotation of the propeller, imagine that you are standing behind the boat, looking at the prop. If it is rotating clockwise when forward gear is engaged, it is a right-hand propeller. Of course, if it's rotating counter-clockwise in forward, it's a left-hand propeller.

Almost all modern mechanical gearboxes for small diesel engines (up to 30–40 hp) require right hand propellers although 30 years ago, left hand propellers were more common in Europe. That's one reason why it's so often necessary to change the propellers when you install a new engine.

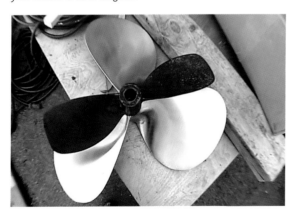

Roobarb's new propeller has a diameter of 16 inches, with three large blades, while the old propeller was a narrow two-blade model with a 13 inch diameter and 10 inch pitch. The new pitch is 11 inches which is slightly more than recommended but is effective, providing 80% of the maximum engine speed is not exceeded.

BUYING A PROPELLER

From the start of this project, my wish list has included a feathering propeller with blades that turn their edges to the water flow and create very little drag when the engine is turned off and you're sailing (and there is no noise from a propeller spinning from the water flow!).

Another option was to buy a folding propeller that also creates little drag when the engine is turned off. I met with the propeller experts from a company that eventually sold me the propeller at a couple of boat shows, and they recommended a conventional three-bladed propeller as the best value-for-money compromise.

A fixed propeller costs much less than a prop with feathering or folding blades, and with no internal moving parts, requires less maintenance. The drawback is that the drag created by a stationary fixed prop will reduce boat speed by parts of a knot. There's always a compromise when selecting boat equipment.

Keeping the old two-blade propeller was not an option, both because it was left-handed and also not configured to transmit the full power of the new engine. Having only two blades minimizes the drag created by a fixed blade prop but can increase vibration on a long-keeled boat since each blade is 'hidden' behind the keel twice every revolution, with a momentary reduction in thrust.

The new three-blade prop I purchased for the boat has much more combined blade area than the old two blade prop – now *Roobarb* powers along like a little tugboat.

Another thing I've noticed is that *Roobarb's* handling has improved. It's never easy to go astern with a long-keeled, single screw boat and *Roobarb* used to turn to port in reverse, no matter which way the rudder was facing. The extra power now makes it easier to compensate for this 'prop-walk' and I can move the throttle and gearshift with confidence that I won't lose control. Or could it be that I'm just getting better at handling her?

BIGGER THAN EXPECTED

The propeller specialists used a computer program to calculate the settings for a propeller – and then applied their experience and judgment to recommend a different prop with a slightly larger diameter. There

Boat talk

Simmer rings: Shaft seals (actually a brand name product made by Simrit). Also called seal rings or radial seals.

Drive train: The assembly of engine, gearbox, couplings and shaft that transfers power from the engine to the propeller.

was plenty of room in the prop aperture and I prefer to run at fairly low prop speeds with plenty of reserve power and acceleration. To simplify the discussion at the prop shop, I'd printed out photographs of the propeller aperture, and then written dimensions on the photographs.

Using a computer program, the experts determined that I needed a 15 inch diameter propeller with 11 inches of pitch, but after I showed him the photos illustrating how big the prop aperture was, John recommended a 16 inch prop with 11 inches of pitch. He told me that the larger blade area would give better power transfer and less propeller slip (a propeller's inefficiency in the water). The recommended prop would be more than enough to get *Roobarb* to hull speed (on a displacement hull the max speed – a function of the waterline length). For *Roobarb* the water line of 7 metres (6.99 metres to be exact) results in a theoretical hull speed of 6.5 knots.

Calculating the theoretical maximum speed of a displacement (non-planing) hull:

Velocity = 2.46 x the square root of the waterline length in meters.

$$v = 2.46\sqrt{LWL}$$

When determining the size of the propeller, the clearance between the blade tips, the hull and the rudder must also be correct. Prop clearances are often tight on small boats (not, however on *Roobarb*) and compromises have to be made regarding diameter and pitch in order to get a reasonably functional combination of those two characteristics. There are rules of thumb for how large the clearance dimensions should be and a good propeller salesman will help you with these. The engine manufacturers

usually want the engine to work well along the whole power curve (range of power outputs) and to be able to reach its maximum recommended speed in rpm. Because I'm careful with engine speed and run my engine to conserve fuel, I chose to heed the advice regarding a propeller with a slightly larger diameter, to get some more drive in headwinds and waves. Perhaps also to get off a lee shore, should it ever be necessary. Installing the propeller itself was one of the easiest jobs.

It's a good idea to put some waterproof grease between the propeller and the shaft – it makes it easier to remove the propeller when necessary. It's essential to have a good propeller puller – one that will fit in the space around the propeller – on hand for this job. Read more in the guide to propeller pullers.

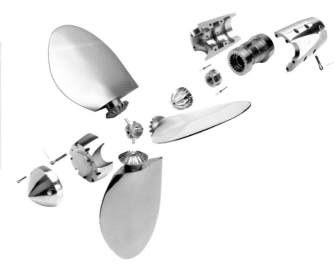

A Maxprop with feathering blades creates little drag when you're sailing. The price for the correct size of this excellent product for Roobarb was close to £2,200 / $3,500, Maxprops are very attractive to boatyard thieves.

PROPELLER SHAFT

I bought a new shaft made from a duplex stainless steel, with a tapered end, since the old one was worn in the section that went through the stuffing box. It didn't make sense to re-use the old shaft when all the other drive train components had been replaced. The cost of the shaft wasn't a large part of the total cost of replacing the engine, especially as the key-less connection of the Bullflex flexible coupling allowed me to buy a standard, one metre length of 25 mm shaft and cut it to the right length (approx. 90 cm, which is quite short for a sailing boat). I did this with an angle grinder, and there was no need for additional machining.

There are several standards used around the world for the taper angle, keyway width and depth and thread gauge at the propeller end of a shaft. It's quite likely that your old shaft does not have the same taper and keyway as your new propeller, so it probably makes sense to buy a new propeller and a new shaft at the same time.

SHAFT LOG

Roobarb had a traditional, 30 year old shaft log made by a local firm for the Yanmar YS-engines. I thought I would have to buy a whole new shaft log but found a newly made replacement bearing at the propeller shop, with the result that I kept the existing tube and saved some money and a lot of trouble and time on the installation.

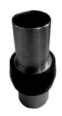

Roobarb's traditional shaft log was fitted with a new water-lubricated rubber bearing (a cutless bearing) and I didn't need to change the log as originally planned. (The shaft log is the tube in the hull around the shaft.)

FLEXIBLE COUPLING

An engine-gearbox assembly standing on flexible mounts moves, while the shaft to which the assembly is attached cannot move, because the shaft must pass through the hull at the shaft log, with bearings at the log and the strut (if a strut is fitted). For this reason – the need to attach something that moves to something that cannot follow that movement – it is desirable to insert flexing devices in the drive train. Traditionally, shaft to gearbox connections have been rigid, but today there is every reason to include a flexible connection, making the installation easier and less sensitive to alignment problems.

A flexible shaft coupling with its strong rubber core has several advantages. The first is that is reduces vibration, especially that originating from fluctuations in engine and shaft speed that resonate through the hull. The other big advantage of a flexible coupling is that it can absorb a couple of degrees of misalignment, so that you don't need to spend hours trying to adjust the engine mounts to the nearest tenth of a mm, while the hull may be flexing under you. This doesn't mean that you don't need to try for perfect alignment –

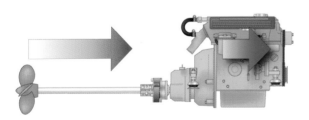

A flexible coupling takes up some of the relative movement between the engine and shaft, and also absorbs small variations in engine power output. These couplings reduce the amount of engine vibration transferred to the hull, increasing comfort and reducing noise.

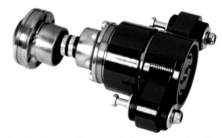

This CV shaft coupling and thrust bearing from Aquadrive absorbs vibration and allows an angled connection between the gearbox and the shaft. Mechanically, the coupling can take up to eight degrees at each of its two CV joints (16 degrees in all) but the recommended ideal arrangement is a maximum of three degrees at each CV joint, to reduce wear.

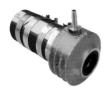

There are several types of shaft seal on the market, each working in its own way to keep water out of the boat. These include radial seals and simmer rings.

the main purpose of a flexible coupling is to take up movement between the shaft and engine when they're both turning, not to permit sloppy installation work. The Vetus Bullflex shaft coupling, which I installed as a part of the repower project, can absorb up to two degrees of misalignment.

The Bullflex coupling made the engine installation considerably faster because the coupling's broad face plate made it easy to see if it was perfectly parallel to the face of the gearbox drive flange. My only problem was getting a torque wrench into the space available to tighten the bolts properly.

CONSTANT VELOCITY SHAFT COUPLINGS (CV JOINTS)

An alternative to a flexible coupling is a constant velocity (CV) coupling, consisting of two CV joints connected by a short shaft, combined with a thrust bearing attached to the hull of the boat. CV joints were developed in the auto industry, and if you have a front wheel drive car, there are four CV joints down there, at each end of both stub axles, connecting your car's gearbox to the front wheels.

The CV joints and the thrust bearing take up relative movement between the gearbox and the prop shaft, and allow the engine-gearbox assembly and shaft to be out of alignment by up to about 16 degrees. This means that the engine can sit level in the boat.

With the engine sitting level there will be an angled connection at the coupling between the gearbox drive flange and the propeller shaft. The thrust bearing is attached to the hull and takes up all the fore and aft forces (thrust) from the propeller, so none of that load is transferred to the engine and its mounts.

An advantage of this is that you can select softer engine mounts which will transmit less vibration to the hull. Unfortunately, a CV coupling adds to the overall length of the shaft – about 250 mm/10 inches for the smallest models. A CV coupling with no keyway required on the shaft will make it easy to cut the shaft to take up this extra length.

SHAFT SEALING

To stop water leaking into a boat through the tube in the hull around the shaft (the shaft log), a seal must be made. Traditionally this has been done with a bronze stuffing box, with waxed or greased fibre packing (usually woven flax) packed around the shaft, to close the gap between the shaft and the bronze body of the stuffing box. These seals drip water continuously to lubricate the contact face between the shaft and the packing. From time to time it's necessary to tighten the gland nut of the stuffing box a little to compress the packing, so as to slow, but not stop, the water drip. For this type of seal to work well, the shaft must be very smooth – any burrs or other irregularities in the shaft will damage the packing. Low friction Teflon packing is now available for stuffing boxes and receives mixed reviews.

Checking a shaft for straightness is best done at the propeller shop. The shaft is supported on rollers, while an index gauge rides on the centre of the shaft, registering any bend or wobble. The allowable tolerance is 0.05 mm per metre for a straight shaft.

The theory behind it all

Let's start with the basics. How fast will the propeller turn? You take the max number of engine revolutions and divide by the gearbox reduction ratio.

For example 3,600 engine revolutions per minute (rpm) transmitted into a 2:1 gearbox results in a shaft speed of 3,600/2 = 1,640 rpm. We also need to know the output (in kW or hp) of the engine, the desired or maximum speed of the boat, the resistance to movement (drag) caused by the shape and surface texture of the hull, the shaft diameter and the space available for the propeller between the end of the shaft, the front of the rudder, and the surrounding elements of the hull (propeller aperture).

>> STEP-BY-STEP

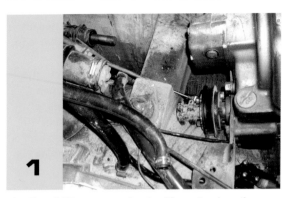

1

▲ The old Yanmar engine had been in place for over 30 years. There was already a flexible shaft coupling that had probably been flexible once but not any longer.

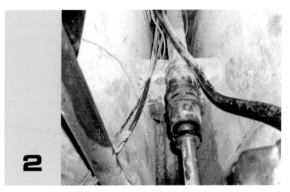

2

▲ The old shaft seal had worked well for a long time. It had worn grooves into the shaft but there hadn't been much leakage.

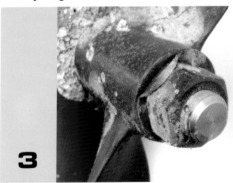

3

▲ The old propeller, a two blade model 13 inches in diameter which, combined with a worn-out engine, didn't provide enough thrust for this heavy boat.

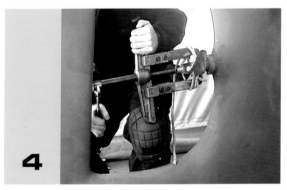

4

▲ The prop was stuck fast and the puller that I had borrowed was a bit too big to grip the propeller.

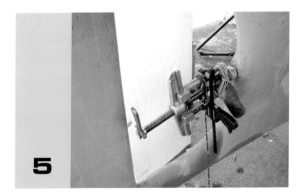

5

▲ Nothing happened despite my efforts. I tried to bind the jaws of the puller together but they kept sliding off the prop. No success, much frustration.

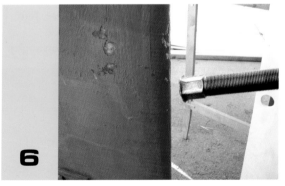

6

▲ As a last resort, I heated the prop with a blow torch and used a hammer to the back of the puller. It worked great in spite of the limited space to swing the hammer between the puller and the rudder skeg.

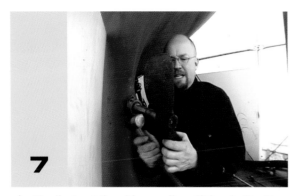

7

▲ Finally, I got the old propeller off the shaft with careful taps from a hammer.

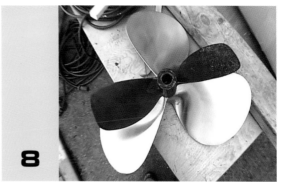

8

▲ There was a considerable difference in size between old and new propellers. I went from a two blade 13 inch to a three blade 16 inch propeller.

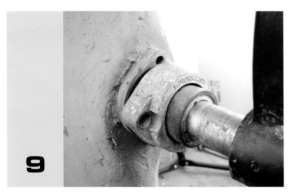

9

▲ In the beginning, I thought I'd have to replace the whole original shaft log and bearing with a new assembly that would include a fibreglass shaft log.

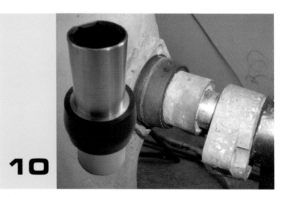

10

▲ Luckily, a newly made original bearing was available as a spare part at the propeller shop, so all I had to do was replace the bearing, which only cost £30/$50.

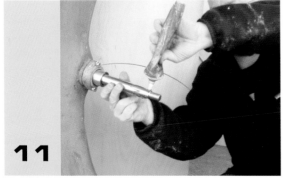

11

▲ The new shaft is getting a layer of marine grease so that it will be easier to remove the propeller next time.

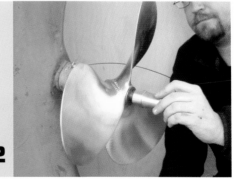

12

▲ A zinc anode was attached to the end of the shaft with a socket head bolt. I bought three extra anodes immediately as my marina has some problems with stray current.

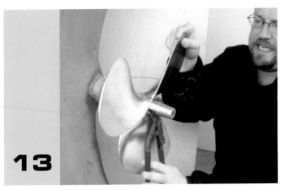

13

▲ The nut on the propeller shaft is tightened (use a proper key wrench) and gets a folding washer for safety.

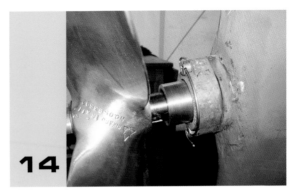

14

▲ The new cutless bearing was in place and the end cap of the shaft log had been seized with stainless steel wire.

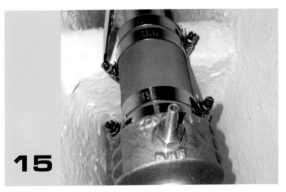

15

▲ The new flexible inner bearing with dual lip seals was held in place by double acid-resistant hose clamps at each end of the flexible tube.

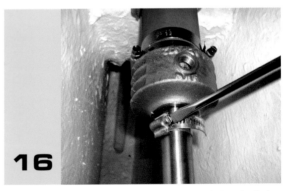

16

▲ A hose clamp was tightened around the shaft for safety, to stop it sliding out of the boat and into the sea in the event of the shaft to gearbox connection failing.

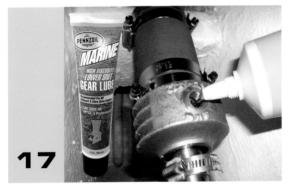

17

▲ Hypoid gear oil (SAE 80W-90) being poured into the shaft seal housing. A plastic tube used as a final filler and sight gauge made it easy to see when the seal housing was full.

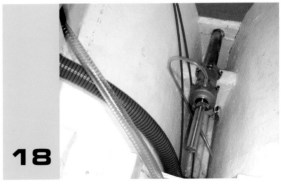

18

▲ The installation of the propeller shaft and seals was complete. The clear plastic sight gauge tube was eventually secured on a bulkhead in plain view.

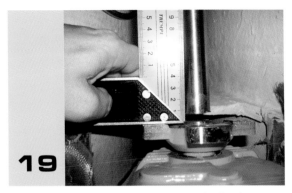

19

▲ In order to fit perfectly, the shaft had to be shortened by 10 cm, to bring it to 90 cm. I cut it with an angle grinder.

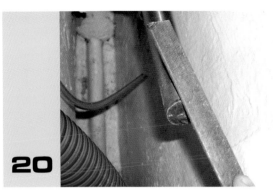

20

▲ The burrs on the cut end of the shaft were removed with a hand file.

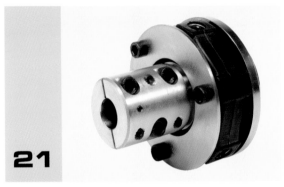

21

▲ A flexible shaft coupling takes up small errors in alignment but more importantly, stops vibration and noise from being transferred to the hull.

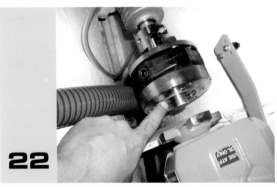

22

▲ After some adjustment of the engine mounts, the flange of the flexible coupling was perfectly parallel with the drive flange of the gearbox. Finally, the engine, gearbox and shaft were aligned!

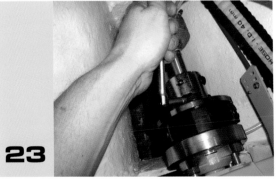

23

▲ Finally, I checked that everything was tightened up, although the final adjustments to the drive train were made when all the other systems were completed and the boat was back in the water as the shape of the hull will be slightly different.

PROJECT LOG

LEVEL OF DIFFICULTY: Easy

TIME SPENT: 10 hours

TOOLS: In order to remove old equipment, you may need to borrow, buy or make special tools. A torque wrench is needed to correctly bolt up the gearbox drive flange to the shaft coupling. In addition to the special tools, you'll need the usual wrenches, spanners, screwdrivers, etc. from your toolbox.

Shaft couplings

A flexible shaft coupling is the best way to connect an engine that twitches on its mounts in response to torque and thrust to a propeller shaft that passes through bearings that are rigidly attached to the hull. The transmission of vibration and noise to the hull is greatly reduced. Another benefit of a flexible coupling is that it can take up small errors in the alignment of the engine-gearbox assembly and the shaft.

The main function of a flexible coupling is to transfer torque from the engine to the shaft, but both radial and axial force fluctuations are also smoothed out, reducing vibration. Some couplings incorporate a thrust bearing, which is rigidly attached to the hull, providing a more efficient transmission of power and less stress on the engine mounts than a continuous shaft arrangement.

Here are three common shaft couplings:

RIGID SHAFT CONNECTION

This is not ideal for a small leisure boat. There are several disadvantages when you compare this approach with the modern alternatives that are available.

FLEXIBLE SHAFT COUPLING

Flexible couplings have rubber or plastic parts that absorb vibrations and minor misalignment (up to a couple of degrees). These couplings are available in a number of different models.

CV-JOINT COUPLING

CV stands for 'Constant Velocity' and this type of power connection, developed in the auto industry, means that the engine and shaft don't have to be aligned at all. A typical marine CV coupling has two CV joints , and works best if the shaft angles are the same on both sides of the assembly, for example 2 x 8 degrees. Having only one of the CV joints angled reduces strength and transmission smoothness, but is the normal situation in marine applications.

In addition to the CV joints, this shaft coupling incorporates a thrust bearing that is rigidly attached to the hull. The thrust bearing performs the vital role of transferring the thrust from the propeller directly to the hull instead of that thrust passing through the gearbox and engine to the engine mounts and from them to the hull. As they no longer have to transfer thrust, the engine mounts can be softer than with a continuous shaft, and these softer mounts will transmit less engine vibration and noise to the hull. All angled connections in the drive train are prone to wear, so it's prudent to run the engine at somewhat reduced power and speed (rpm's) with such connections. In addition to the added cost of the CV couplings, there is often a problem with space, as the shortest couplings with CV joints are around 25 cm long.

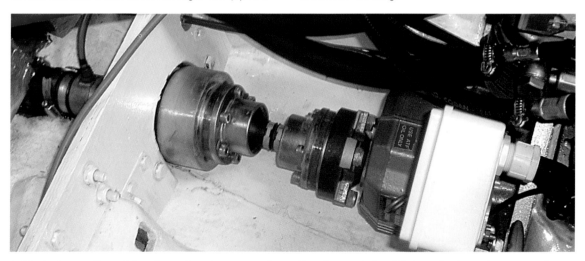

A CV shaft coupling with a thrust bearing can reduce vibration and simplify installation of a new engine. I could unfortunely not fit one in Roobarb, as there was not enough space.

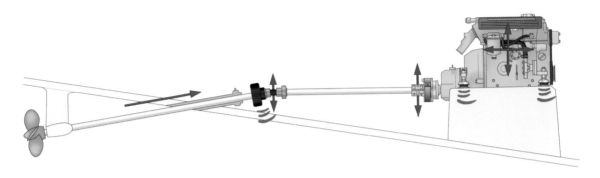

This sketch shows the different forces that affect the drive train, and illustrates with red arcs the main points where noise is transferred to the hull. With a CV coupling the engine can be installed level, making the installation easier and improving the engine's internal lubrication.

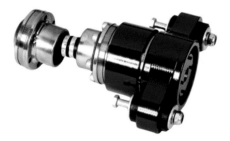

Aquadrive couplings were developed from the original Scatra couplings. Unicardan developed the first Aquadrive coupling in1977.

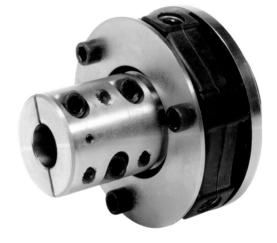

A flexible shaft-coupling, like the Vetus Bullflex shown here, reduces the vibration and misalignment that occur when the engine and hull move relative to each other. This coupling can also centre the shaft on the gearbox drive flange.

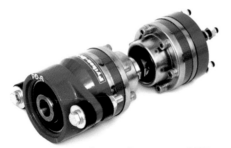

There are now several manufacturers of CV couplings with integral thrust bearings, including Python-Drive, Hydra-Drive and Vetus. Some of these competitors may be less expensive than the Aquadrive products in different markets.

FOCUS SELECTING THE RIGHT PROPELLER

Traditionally, the configuration of the propeller has been calculated with a nomogram chart and a measure of experience. Today a computer program is used – and a measure of experience.

When you go to buy a propeller, the salesman will ask questions about the type of boat, the hull, the power output and speed (rpm's) of the engine, the size of the propeller aperture, the expected speed of the boat, and, of course, your budget.

The salesman or a technician enters this information into the computer to generate calculated recommendations, and then uses his experience to interpret those recommendations and select the best propeller for your boat and your budget.

If you want to have a go at propeller selection yourself, there are free programs on the web, including Propeller Pitch at www.castlemarine. co.uk/pitch.htm. A Google or Yahoo search will find other propeller software.

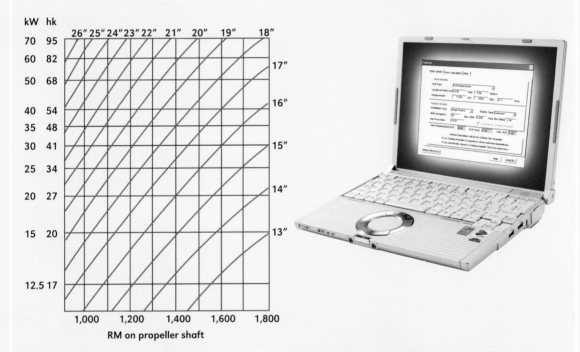

Nomogram on which you can cross reference engine output and shaft speed to find recommended prop size.

The program Propeller Pitch Calculator can be downloaded from the Internet so that you can test the numbers yourself. A recommendation will then appear regarding which propeller is likely to be a good choice. Bear in mind that a computer program can't replace an expert – there is no substitute for experience.

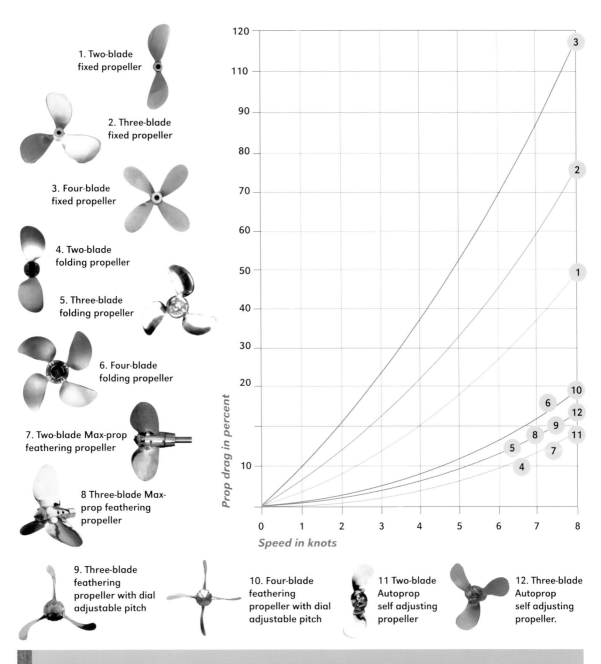

1. Two-blade fixed propeller

2. Three-blade fixed propeller

3. Four-blade fixed propeller

4. Two-blade folding propeller

5. Three-blade folding propeller

6. Four-blade folding propeller

7. Two-blade Max-prop feathering propeller

8 Three-blade Max-prop feathering propeller

9. Three-blade feathering propeller with dial adjustable pitch

10. Four-blade feathering propeller with dial adjustable pitch

11 Two-blade Autoprop self adjusting propeller

12. Three-blade Autoprop self adjusting propeller.

WATER RESISTANCE CREATED BY SAILBOAT PROPELLERS
This graph from the Dutch research company Amartech shows the water resistance or drag created by several common propellers used on sailing boats. The tests were made in a pool and the base line for the values was the water resistance of a non-rotating three-blade fixed propeller being pulled through the water at 9 knots. Hull and rudder shape, and their effect on water flow around the boat, may cause the actual effect of prop drag to vary from one boat to another. See www.amartech.nl

FOCUS   DIFFERENT TYPES OF PROPELLERS

FIXED BLADE PROPELLERS

Fixed propellers for sailboats are most often two- or three-bladed. For sail boats/motor boats there are propellers with four, five or more blades. Traditionally, sailing boats have had two-bladed, fixed propellers.

Replacing an old engine with a new one frequently results in increased power output. To provide adequate propeller blade area to use that power in the limited aperture space between the shaft, the hull and the rudder, you may have to go for more blades and more pitch on a prop with the same diameter as the old prop.

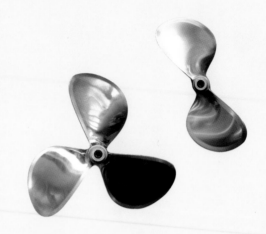

FEATHERING PROPELLERS

A feathering propeller turns its almost flat blades edge on to the water stream in order to minimize the drag of the prop when sailing. A feathering prop usually has more blade area than a folding propeller of the same diameter. The pitch of a feathering prop can be changed, either after disassembling the prop or in some cases adjusting an external dial. There are models, notably the Autoprop, with swinging blades with complex shapes and curvatures that automatically adjust themselves, effectively changing diameter and pitch, or feathering, to suit shaft revolutions and boat speed.

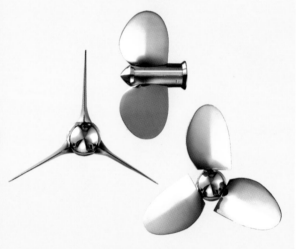

FOLDING PROPELLERS

The blades of a folding propeller close back in line with the shaft when rotation stops, and open out by centrifugal force when shaft rotation starts. The first folding props appeared more than thirty years ago, as a simple way to reduce drag when sailing, but they've come a long way since then, with increased efficiency and more ability to function in reverse – not thought of as a strong point for folding props.

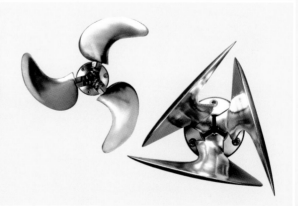

COMPARISON OF DIFFERENT PROPELLERS

Type of propeller	Benefits	Drawbacks
Fixed blade	• large blade area • relatively inexpensive	• high water resistance/drag can considerably lower the speed of a boat under sail
Feathering	• a large blade area • works equally well in forward or reverse • has low drag/water resistance when sailing	• more expensive than a fixed blade prop • less efficient compared to a fixed propeller
Folding	• low drag/water resistance when sailing	• reduced efficiency and slow engagement in reverse

OTHER PROPELLERS

There's a wide variety of propellers types, working in slightly different ways and made from a range of materials but the types mentioned above are the most common for the recreational sailing boats that I discuss in this book.

It's interesting to think about the future of the propeller, when it may not have a hub in the centre but instead have blades rooted along an outer ring. The theoretical advantage is that this arrangement results in less disturbed water, with more energy going into thrust, and less into radial water movement.

MATERIAL

Most propellers are made from a bronze, such as manganese bronze and nickel aluminium bronze. Bronze is an alloy of copper and tin, with other metals frequently added to enhance its performance in different applications. Bronze has a low melting point, is relatively hard and lends itself well to casting. Propellers are also made of stainless steel, composites containing glass fibre, carbon fibre and thermoplastics.

A metal propeller should normally be protected by a sacrificial anode, most commonly zinc in salt water and aluminium in fresh and brackish water. Some research shows that zinc anodes can increase the rate of organic fouling, barnacles in particular, on bronze propellers under water. Not enough research is made in this field yet, to be certain.

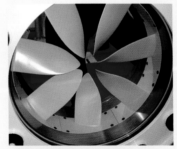

A new developed type of propeller that we may see even on recreational boats in the future.

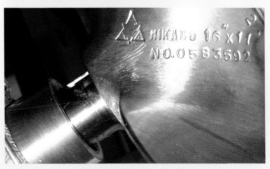

The size of a propeller is given with two numbers, for example 16 x 11. The first number, 16, gives the diameter in inches; the second is the pitch in inches (1 inch = 25.4 mm).

FOCUS SHAFT SEALS

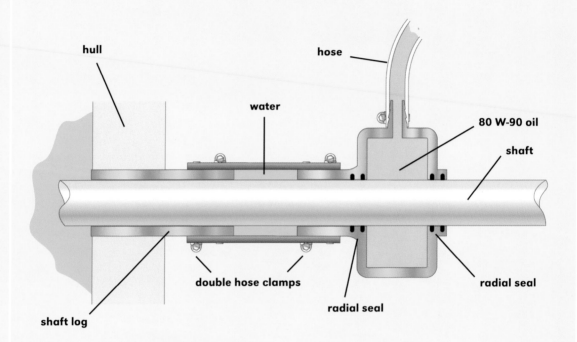

hull

hose

water

80 W-90 oil

shaft

double hose clamps

radial seal

radial seal

shaft log

A shaft seal works on the principle that a flexible material, in a housing or case close to a bearing, encircles the shaft, in firm but not tight contact with it, and stops water getting into the boat through the gap between the shaft and the shaft log tube.

There are four main types of shaft seal that keep the water out of the boat:

- traditional tallow/grease packing stuffing boxes (that drip water)
- oil- or water-lubricated radial seals
- water-lubricated axial seals
- dripless seals consisting of a stainless steel ring, attached to the shaft, that seals against a static ring of graphite or silicon mounted on a stainless steel tube attached to one end of a corrugated rubber pipe, itself, clamped to the inboard end of the shaft log

For *Roobarb* I chose an oil-lubricated shaft seal assembly with radial seals of a simple and inexpensive type recommended by the engine dealer.

It's worth remembering that shaft seals wear out and that there is a recommended maximum time between replacements for each type. As most of the old stuffing boxes with flax and tallow have been in place for 20–30 years on many boats, the life span of a new shaft seal is not a big worry.

Most modern shaft seal assemblies are flexible, with a short length of marine hose attached to the inboard end of the shaft log. This allows the seal to follow any radial movements of the shaft resulting from misalignment or being slightly bent. Too much of this wobbling movement can cause premature failure of the seal and the shaft bearings, so you still need to focus on having a straight and properly-aligned shaft.

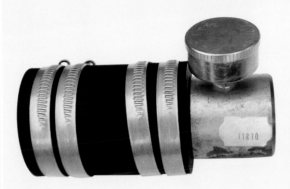

The traditional model, lubricated with grease, is common on older boats. Often the grease cap is connected to a grease injector and needs to be twisted a notch after each voyage. It will also drip slightly.

A dripless seal is a water-lubricated shaft seal in which the actual seal is made between the faces of a stainless steel ring attached to the shaft and a stator ring of graphite indirectly attached to the shaft log. These seals create no wear on the shaft and are essentially maintenance free. Lubricating water is supplied from an intake scoop.

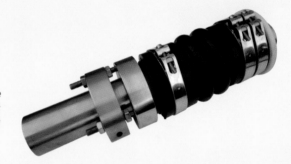

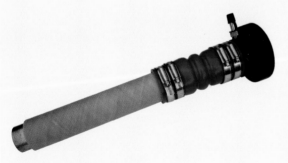

A radial or 'lip' seal assembly has a seal housing made of a composite plastic. The seals can be changed without completely removing the shaft from the boat. Lip seals are lubricated by water from the raw water system of the engine, or from a separate sea water intake scoop on the hull.

A simple shaft seal assembly with a bronze case holding double, oil lubricated, rotary shaft seals (Simmer rings). This was the type of shaft seal installed on Roobarb during the repower project and is one of the most frequently used shaft sealing methods in all kinds of machinery...

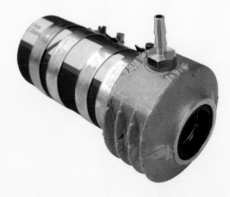

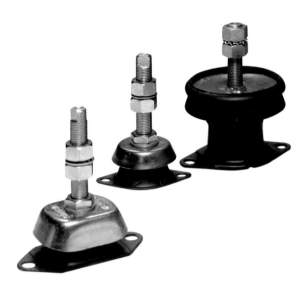

Engine mountings

Engine mountings are also called engine mounts, engine isolators, engine feet and even engine cushions. Whatever the name, they are the inboard engine's attachment to the engine bed and hull.

Their most important functions are to hold the engine in place, resist the torque from the shaft on the engine-gearbox assembly (for every action, an equal and opposite reaction), and unless there's a thrust bearing in the drive train, transfer the thrust developed by the prop to the hull. In addition, the flexibility of the engine mounts also dampens the transmission of engine vibration to the hull, reducing noise and increasing comfort.

Several large forces affect the engine mounts. In addition to supporting the weight of the engine, they are under the influence of the axial force or thrust from the propeller shaft when the engine is in gear and working to move the boat, ahead or astern. As mentioned, the mounts also resist the torque that wants to turn the engine around with the same force that rotates the axle.

The engine and its attachments are also impacted when a boat goes into a wave or trough – the force of the vertical acceleration and deceleration can be considerable, with G-forces increasing the load on the engine mounts as much as eightfold. To say the least, the engine mountings take a lot of punishment!

There is a wide variety of engine mountings to suit the conditions and manner in which the boat will be operated. They are made from rubber or synthetic compounds formulated for their load-carrying and vibration-dampening characteristic.

The basic construction of an engine mount includes a flexible rubber core, sandwiched between upper and lower metal half-shells. To eliminate the possibility of a very heavy or powerful engine breaking free of its mounts, as might occur in a deep roll or capsize, with the risk of damage to the hull and injury to the crew, the steel bearer bolts of some engine mounts pass through the rubber core and are secured under the lower shell, which is in turn bolted to the engine beds of the hull.

The rubber in the engine mounts takes on a permanent set or deformation quite quickly, so the engine-gearbox assembly and shaft need to be adjusted for alignment after a couple of weeks of running-in a new engine or a new set of mounts.

After a couple of years, the engine mountings will have compressed further, and another re-alignment will be in order. After 8–12 years, the mounts need to be replaced – they are consumables that wear out.

The flexible part of a mounting is often based on natural rubber which is damaged by oil and other chemicals, so don't let oil or diesel drip or spill on to the mountings, and wipe them clean frequently.

Get the recommendations of the manufacturer's salesman or technician if you don't have a clear understanding of which engine mounts will work best on your boat. If possible, get oil-dampened mountings.

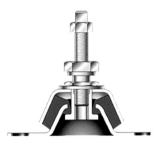

A block of rubber is here glued between the two metal half-shells. If the rubber rips apart, the half-shells of a mount must still stay together, so that the engine cannot break loose, endangering the boat and crew.

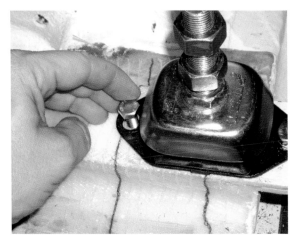

The engine mount base plates/lower half-shells often have elongated bolt holes. Using high tensile hold-down bolts that are a couple of millimetres smaller in diameter than the holes, allows some room for adjustment. When the engine is positioned on the beds and before the hold-down bolts are installed, the base plates of the mounts must be flat to the engine beds and parallel to the long axis of the engine so that no bending stresses develop in the bolts or the engine legs as the bolts are tightened down. You can check that each mount is correctly positioned before bolting by lifting the engine slightly with a crowbar to let the rubber of the mount return to its original shape and the base plate move to its unstressed position. (More about this in Chapter 8.)

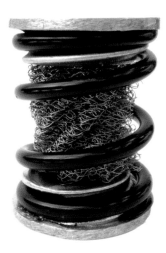

An isolator from Aquamer with a steel spring and a damping core of stainless steel 'wool'. An engine stabilizer bar is frequently used in conjunction with these mounts.

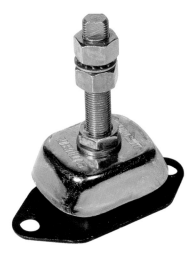

At the recommendation of my engine technician support, the Vetus KSTEUN 75 mounts for Roobarb's engine are one size larger than the engine manufacturer's specification.

A tip from the expert

I met an experienced technician from the Jachtwerf Daniël company with may engine installations under his belt, and he strongly suggested to use viscous hydro-damper mountings. They are oil-filled hydraulic shock absorbers that prevent the engine starts to wobble from the forces from the shaft rotation and movements in waves.

Unfortunately these mountings were too tall to fit into *Roobarb* without even more modification of the engine bed.

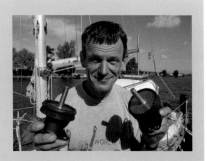

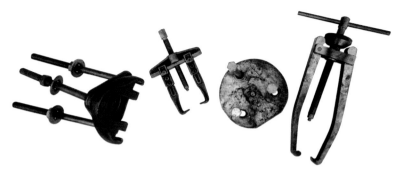

A variety of pullers that the propeller specialist may need to have in the tool box.

Propeller pullers

It can be difficult to remove an old propeller that has been tight on its shaft for many years.

A prop puller with three claws for a three-bladed prop, or two claws for a two-blade prop, is the tool needed for this job. There are not many purpose-made prop pullers available in general tool stores, automotive gear pullers being more common, so propeller manufacturers often make their own pullers. Short term, the least expensive approach is to borrow a puller for the job in progress, but a puller is an essential tool for the do-it-yourself boat owner, who may need to replace a damaged prop on a long cruise. You can make your own puller – a home-made model, with triangular side plates and long bolts, is shown in the collection at the top of this page, and if you're not a metalworker, you can use plywood for the side plates, although they may need to frequent replacement.

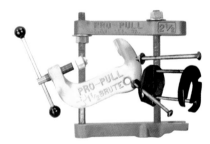

Some of the commercial pullers on the market.

GENTLE FORCE

Trying to remove a prop by hammering it off is not a good idea – it's likely to damage the prop and in the worst case, may also damage the shaft and bearings. Most of the time, it's only possible to hit the hub of the prop on one side at a time, so the hammering force is off-centre and likely to jam the prop even harder onto the shaft.

It often helps to heat up the hub of the prop with a blowtorch for a minute or two, but be careful to keep the flame moving, so that the hub expands uniformly and so that you don't melt or oxidize a weak spot into the metal, and of course, don't get the flame on or near a good cutlass bearing. The hub will expand enough to make it much easier to pull the prop off, just remember how hot it is and wear thick work-gloves when you're setting up and working the puller.

PULLER PROBLEMS

The puller that I borrowed and used to remove *Roobarb*'s old propeller was far too big for the job and the claws didn't grab and set well. It kept sliding sideways and slipping off the prop as I tightened the pusher bolt. I tried binding the claws with clamps and rope, but to no avail; they still slipped.

After struggling with this for quite a while, I changed tacks, heated the hub and hit the back of the spreader bar of the puller hard with a hammer, as close as I could get to the pusher bolt to keep the force near center, and the prop finally came off. Phew!

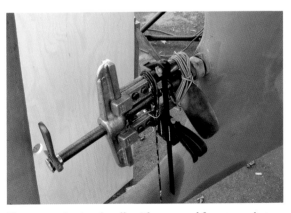

The wrongly sized puller I borrowed for removing the old propeller on Roobarb.

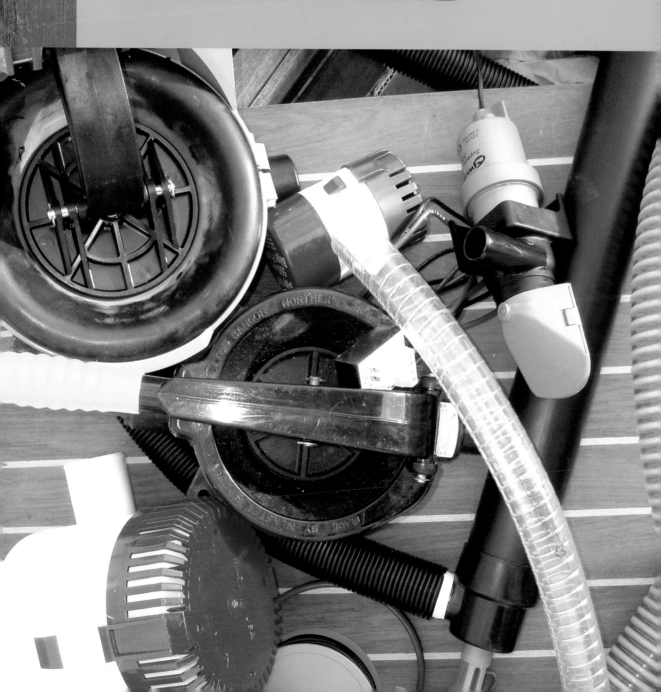

06
BILGE PUMPS AND FILTERS

THE PUMPS THAT SAVE THE BOAT

A high quality, high capacity bilge pump – or better still, several high quality, high capacity bilge pumps – are among the most important items of security equipment on board.
While not in the same league as bilge pumps, good filters reduce the risk of failure for all the boat systems they protect, including the engine, and discharge filters keep the waters clean.

We'll now take a close look at two installations and review what needs to be considered when assembling a system. From my own experience, I think that the hardest part of installing a bilge pump is finding a good place for it. On a modern boat there is often a sump for the bilge pump, but on the project boat *Roobarb*, I had to simply locate the pumps in the lowest part of the bilge, a place under the engine with poor accessibility. I tried to improve things by installing some removable stainless steel pump access plates, but servicing those pumps is always going to be a difficult job.

That's why I have several back-ups should the main pump fail – five all-told, in addition to some buckets and the emergency possibility of letting the engine's impeller pump suck water from the inside of the boat.

EVERY BOAT SHOULD HAVE AT LEAST ONE BILGE PUMP

Anything other than the smallest of recreational boats should have at least one automatic bilge pump, controlled by a float switch or other water level sensor that turns on the pump as soon as the water in the bilge reaches a certain level. This bilge pump should be connected directly to a battery bank, so that the pump works even when the main switch is turned off, as might be the case when the boat is moored or docked.

The second line of defence in a bilge pump system is a big pump that can move a lot of water in the event of a major leak.

All hoses need to be reinforced with a spiral winding of wire or synthetic filament. Low cost hose may kink in a tight bend and impede the water flow. It may also deform as it is softened by the heat of the engine.

A hole in the hull, 30 cm/1 foot below the water line and just the size of the palm of your hand, will let in more than 3,300 litres/870 US gallons of water per minute. To keep up with that much flooding is impossible even for a large, battery-powered bilge pump, but such a pump does give the crew a little more time to find and plug a leak before the boat sinks. Mechanical pumps driven by their own engines can handle heavy flooding but they are rarely carried on board small boats.

CAPACITY

The stated capacity of most bilge pumps is given at zero head, as though the intake and discharge points are at the same level as the pump; this does not correspond to reality on a boat. In most recreational boats, the bilge water has to be lifted 1–2 metres/3–6 feet and this considerably reduces the volume of water actually pumped. A halving of the capacity is typical when the water has to be lifted is a couple of metres and one metre's, lift will reduce the capacity by 25%.

HOSES

It's desirable for water hoses to be reinforced with spiral winding. This is most often accomplished with steel wire for rubber hoses, and with nylon filament for clear plastic tubing. To maintain an unrestricted flow the inside of these pipes must be smooth, as a corrugated lining can reduce water flow at a given

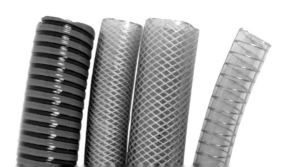

Water flow calculation

You can calculate the approximate amount of water flowing through a broken skin fitting/through hull fitting or a hole made by grounding (1 dm², 30 cm under the waterline), using the following formula, which gives water flow in cubic metres per hour (a cubic metre is 1,000 litres of water or 264 US gallons).

Water flow: $3,600 \times k \times F \times \sqrt{(2 \times g \times h)}$.

F: size of the hole in square metres.

h: the depth of the hole below the surface in metres.

g: constant 9.81 m/s².

k: conversion factor, approx 0.6 for thin cracks with sharp edges, 0.95 for holes with round edges.

Example: for a 100 mm x 100 mm (4" x 4") = 0.1 m² hole, 30 cm = 0.3 m (1') below the waterline.

$Q = 3,600 \times 0.95 \times 0.1 \times \sqrt{(2 \times 9.81 \times 0.3)}$ = 201.3 m³ = 201,300 litres per hour = 3,350 litres (884 US gallons) per minute.

pressure by as much as one third. To minimize internal surface area and friction, water hoses, especially those from bilge pumps, should be kept as short as possible and clamped in position with gentle bends.

For a sailboat, the bilge pump discharge must be above the water line at all angles of heel. As a safety measure you can set the hose up with a vented high point above the discharge fitting, to prevent back flooding when the boat is rail down, providing that the high point doesn't exceed the maximum lift of the pump. The skin fitting/though-hull for the bilge pump discharge should be thin-walled, with the largest possible internal diameter, to avoid impeding water flow.

Non-return valves/check valves can also reduce water flow considerably but are useful in stopping water from draining back to the sump when the pumps shuts down, which with a small sump and a high lift, can cause the pump to cycle on an off continuously, or at least until it burns out.

ALARMS AND LEVEL CONTROLS

If you have an automatically activated bilge pump, a fairly large leak can go unnoticed, as the sound of the pump is hidden by the noise of the engine and other machinery. This makes it easy to miss that the seal on the propeller shaft is starting to leak, for example. In the worst case, the crew, unaware of a leak, leaves the boat, the bilge pump drains the batteries, the pump stops and the boat sinks at its mooring or dock. One way of ensuring that you know that the pump is running is to insert an audio-visual alarm in the circuit between the pump and its automatic switch.

The most common automatic bilge pump control is a float switch with a metal ball that closes the circuit between two contact points and starts the pump, a function that used to be performed by a mercury switch before the environmental dangers of mercury were properly respected. The weak point of mechanical float switches is that they are sensitive to dirt in the bilge water and can get stuck in the open or closed position.

To control the bilge pump on *Roobarb* we installed a water-level control switch with an integrated microprocessor that measures the electrical resistance of the pump to determine if it is lifting water. This control device cycles the pump at regular intervals and if there is no water to pump, the device stops the pump after a couple of seconds, but if there is water, the pump keeps going until the control switch senses a reduction in resistance. This level control device can be set for different time intervals, from 5–120 minutes, at which to start the pump and measure the resistance.

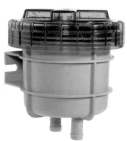

The small bilge pump discharges through a bilge water/oil separator. Over time, these filtering devices are likely to become compulsory everywhere. Already, you can incur large fines in the Eastern Mediterranean and in US waters if you pump anything into the sea other than clean water

THE INSTALLATION

To install a bilge pump is not especially difficult, once you've found a space at the lowest point of the bilge and worked out how to mount the pump there so that it can't move. With that done, all you've got left to do is wire it up. Having said that, I'll go through it step-by-step.

All pumps and automatic switches must be installed so that they are stable. A pump that moves around can suck air, causing the electric motor to race and, if that goes on long enough, burn out.

It's not a good idea to attach a bilge pump by screwing its mounting bracket directly to the hull. If there is no suitable screw base, such as a fibreglass or wooden surface, you will have to make one and glue it in place with an epoxy- or polyurethane-based marine adhesive, such as Sikaflex. The low point of *Roobarb*'s bilge is both deep and hard to reach, located directly under the engine. I had to find an approach that would make it possible to take out the pumps and clean them. After some pondering, I realized that if I glued or screwed the pump mounting brackets at the very bottom of the bilge, it would be very difficult to get them out for cleaning – so the attachments would also have to be removable.

My welder contact helped me to make two stainless pump mounting plates. These long mounts allow the pump to be lifted out of the awkward space under the engine. I was careful to keep the bilge pump discharge hoses as straight as possible, with gentle, wide radius bends.

In connecting the pump and water level control switch to the batteries, great care must be taken at the joints between the wires of the pump and the boat wiring system. While these connections must be tied back to keep them out of the bilge water, they will still be in damp conditions and rarely inspected. Some bilge pumps come with very short wires, further complicating the task of keeping the connections dry.

These, and all other wiring connections on the boat, should be made with marine grade crimped connectors, but these damp environment connections must also protected by heat-shrink insulating tubes of the type that are lined with a thermo glue. Some waterproof crimp fittings are supplied with heat-shrink, glue-lined insulation tubes. Do everything possible to prevent it happening, but when you're making these connections, assume that they're going to end up under water.

FILTERS

Several filters are required for an engine installation. Filters remove dirt from the engine oil and the fuel, and several of them are required for a new engine. There will also be a raw-water filter, called a strainer, mounted close to the raw water intake scoop, to catch

Drawing from experience

On a couple of my earlier boats I've had a couple of close calls, with water above the floorboards. So I've given some thought to how to get an efficient bilge pump system.

The first time I was in, it was the hose-to-skin fitting/through-hull fitting that burst when its contents turned to ice one very cold winter. The boat had been in the water all winter but I discovered the leak in time and had to spend a couple of hours pumping it out – a narrow escape.

On the second occasion, the propeller shaft seal worked loose during the night, in the middle of the wide Pacific, with big seas and strong winds and a long way from nearest island. We couldn't hear where the water was coming in – the source of the leak was already submerged inside the boat, but we eventually found it by feeling around each fitting for water flow. In both cases the boats lacked an automatic bilge pump, and only had manual pumps.

Since I am again equipping a boat for a long-distance cruise, I had been thinking about different solutions and decided to have a good back up to the main bilge pump, to wear both a belt and braces/suspenders on my foul weather gear. I am taking at least five different pumps to empty the boat should the sea reach the wrong side of the hull.

Likely leak locations

Ideally, a boat would not take in any water at all, but in reality a completely dry bilge is a rare thing. If nothing is leaking in from below the water line, rainwater finds a way in from above it, as does seawater from wet decks.

Skin fittings or through hulls, as they are called in North America, are weak points, and a modern boat often has between 5 and 10 (or more) of them. They can break as easily while underway as when moored or docked. The only way of checking them is to have the boat ashore and apply gentle force at each fitting, replacing any that move against the hull or show signs of deterioration. Open and close all valves several times a season to keep them in good working order.

The seal around the propeller shaft protects another opening from the sea, so make sure that you know how it works and how to service it.

Cut-away sterns are a big problem for motor boats with heavy outboard motors. When waves and wakes from passing boats surge over the low transom, the cockpit holds the water, the boat rides lower in the water and is then more susceptible to flooding from the next wave or wake.

Make sure water can't get into the boat through a bilge pump outlet fitting set near the waterline. A check valve or a vented gooseneck in the hose from the pump to the discharge fitting can prevent backflow into the bilge.

---

dirt and debris before it can reach the impeller pump and the rest of the engine cooling system.

A recreation boat like *Roobarb* may also be fitted with air filters to catch odours from the vent lines of fuel tanks and holding tanks, and separator filters to stop oil and grease in bilge water from being pumped overboard.

As previously mentioned, cruising boats may also carry a fuel filter built into a funnel, to check the diesel from a fuel dock before contaminated fuel can get into the boat's tanks. Almost all modern engines have a fuel filter, with an exchangeable, fine grade element, that will catch dirt down to a ten micron particle size (read more about this in the fact box page 89).

A coarser pre-filter, preferably with a water separator function, should always supplement and protect the fine filter mounted on the engine. This primary filter should be easy to empty and service, even in rough conditions, as that's when dirt is stirred up in the tank and fuel-related engine problems start.

If the boat has enough room, a fuel filter assembly with two canisters is a worthwhile upgrade, as it allows a clogged or waterlogged filter to be shut down and serviced without stopping the engine – a great benefit in heavy seas. I installed a single

canister primary fuel filter on *Roobarb* but I'm thinking about upgrading to a two canister model.

CLEANING DIESEL FUEL

In the USA, it is quite common for a tank cleaning company to pump out a big boat's fuel and haul it away for 'polishing' while tank cleaning is in progress. The dirty fuel is taken to a facility where it is run through a series of filters, each finer than the last, to remove sediment, microbes and other contaminants. Some polishing processes also use magnetic fields to recondition the fuel. With the tank cleaned, the polished fuel is pumped back onboard. This is an expensive process but is still less costly than completely replacing a large quantity of fuel.

THE ENVIRONMENT

Almost every boat has a small amount of oil in its bilge, and without discharge filtering, some of that oil goes into the water when the bilge pump operates. This is already a serious offense in the USA and some other countries, and is certain to become one everywhere, as environmental awareness spreads. To prevent this on *Roobarb*, I installed a bilge water filter which reduces the pump capacity quite a bit (I haven't yet made the time to measure the reduction).

FOCUS

QUICK-RELEASE FOR THE SEA WATER PUMP

On the new engine the location of the raw-water impeller pump housing is not well suited to *Roobarb*'s interior arrangements, as it faces away from the person working at the front of the engine. The space is so tight I can't get my head in to see the face plate of the pump.

For a major repair job on the pump, some intervening equipment could be removed to improve access, but that's not something you want to tackle when there are cooling problems at sea. Reaching the nuts while holding the pump face plate with a spanner/open-ended wrench was hard, but to loosen the nuts without dropping them into *Roobarb*'s deep bilge was even harder. I had to find a better way.

My first idea was to insert a metal bowl under the pump to catch anything I dropped, but that was exactly where the hose from the sea water strainer connected to the pump, about 10 cm/ 4 inches away from the skin fitting/through hull.

DO IT YOURSELF

You can buy quick-release kits for impeller pumps in marine accessory shops. These kits contain threaded studs and wing nuts or even new face plates with large thumbscrews. Inspired by the kits I had seen, I made my own for a fraction of the retail price. The job itself was completed in half an hour and cost less than £5/$7. I still expect to drop a wing nut from time to time, so carry a few for the inevitable fumble.

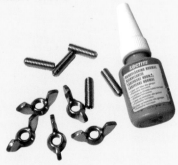

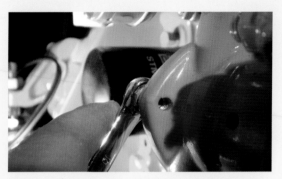

1 To reach the far side of the pump with a spanner/open-ended wrench is hard, and the risk of dropping the nuts is very high.

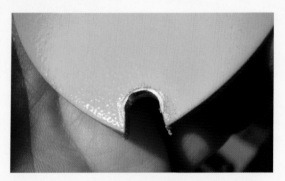

2 I used an angle grinder to open up one of the screw holes into a slot. This is where the first wing nut will engage.

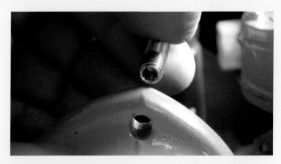

3 All the stud threads were coated with a liquid thread-locking compound, to protect against the studs working loose from the vibration of the engine.

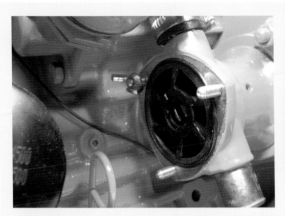

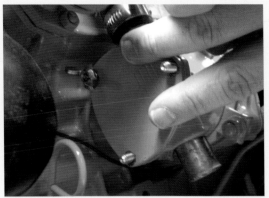

4 The face plate was removed, but it was still difficult to remove the impeller. The camera was wriggled in behind the engine to take this photograph.

5 To reinstall the face plate I put one of the wing nuts on a stud, and then slid the slotted bolt hole of the faceplate under that wing nut and hold the plate while I put on the other two.

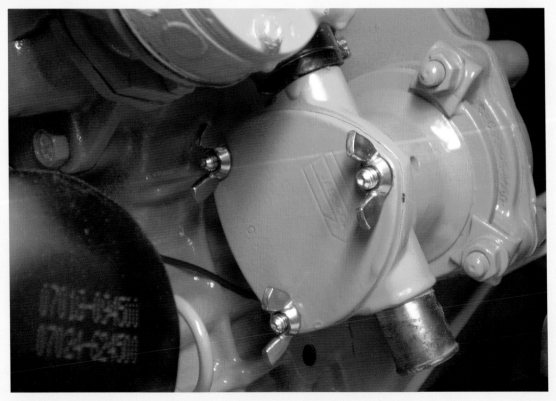

6 With the wing nuts in place it will be easier to replace the impeller in an emergency.

>> STEP-BY-STEP

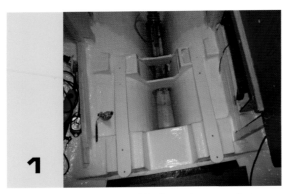

1

▲ With the new engine lifted out, I got ready to install the bilge pump carriers that would end up in the lowest part of the bilge, under the engine.

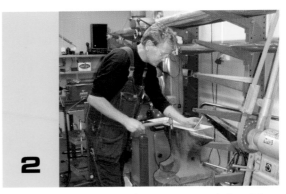

2

▲ To be able to service the pumps I needed stainless steel carriers for them, and asked a machinist and welder to fabricate these plates for me.

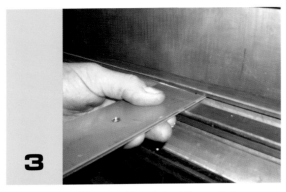

3

▲ He cut and bent acid-resistant 3mm plates according to my measurements. This is a job that's hard to do yourself if you don't have the equipment.

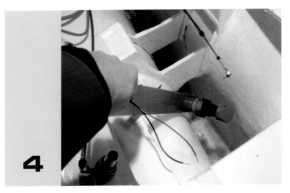

4

▲ The little pump is placed at the lowest point of the bilge. There were several possible locations but I had to make sure that the hose runs would work.

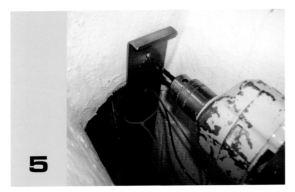

5

▲ I drilled a hole in the stainless steel carrier to fit over the bolt that had been glued into a tapped hole in the hull. A large wing nut will allow the carrier, with the pump attached, to be lifted out without tools.

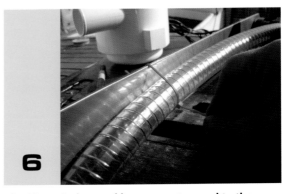

6

▲ The spiral wound hose was strapped to the pump carrier with zip ties and then run in soft bends up the side of the hull to the discharge fitting.

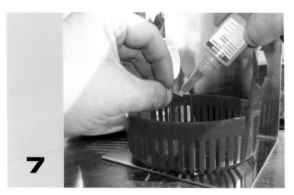

▲ For the big emergency pump, we created a similar carrier to which we attached the bottom of the pump, coating all bolts with thread locking compound.

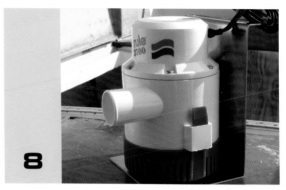

▲ I tapped threaded holes into the base plate of the carrier so that I could bolt through the removable bottom housing of the pump directly to the stainless steel.

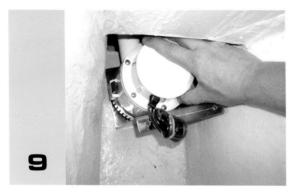

▲ I checked to make sure that I could really get the pump out of the bilge, despite the tight fit. Everything on a boat must be accessible for maintenance.

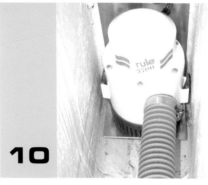

▲ The large emergency pump was in place, 10 cm/4 inches above the bottom of the bilge. This pump will only be used when there is too much water in the bilge for the small pump to handle.

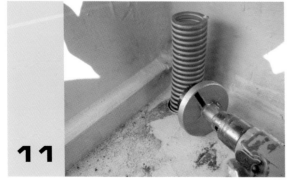

▲ A good hose layout requires a lot of planning – the goal is to have hoses as straight as possible.

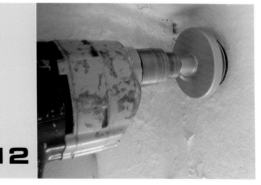

▲ The discharge fitting should be as high as possible on the topsides, to minimize the possibility of the fitting being under water when the boat heels or rolls, as this can result in the bilge pump being back-flooded.

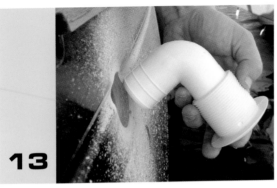

13 ▲ The skin fitting/through-hull penetration was plastic with an integral elbow, so the hose connection would point straight down toward the bilge. The fitting was bedded in a marine grade sealant/caulking.

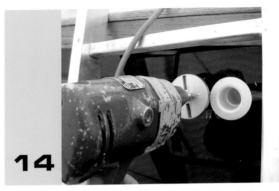

14 ▲ A second penetration was drilled with a hole saw, halfway from the inside, and then half way from the outside, to eliminate surface damage as the saw broke through.

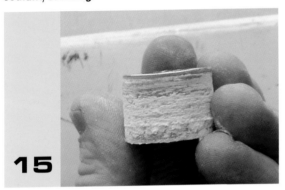

15 ▲ *Roobarb*'s hull thickness is amazing – no wonder the little eight metre boat weighs 4.2 tonnes/9260 pounds.

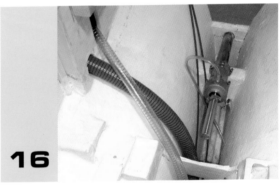

16 ▲ The hoses to the electrically powered bilge pumps are in place. A 38 mm reinforced hose for the manual bilge pump is yet to come.

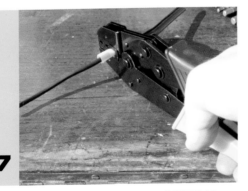

17 ▲ The cables for the pumps are 4 mm²/AWG 11 and are joined with marine-grade, waterproof, crimped butt connectors. Use a rachet crimping tool to get perfect compressed contacts.

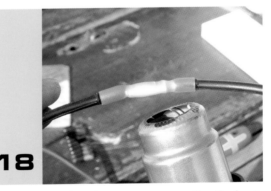

18 ▲ The connections become waterproof as the heat shrink sleeve with its thermo glue lining is carefully warmed with a heat gun.

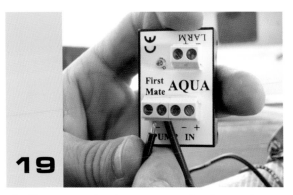

19

▲ The automatic microprocessor level control switch is installed between the battery and the small pump. I set the timer to turn on the pump every 30 minutes.

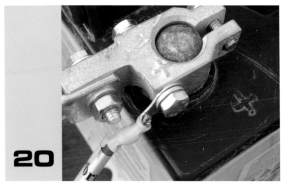

20

▲ The electrical power for the little pump was taken directly from the battery, with a connection to the side lug of the battery terminal.

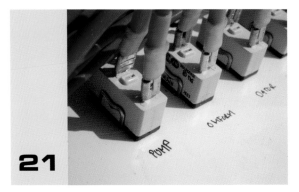

21

▲ The large bilge pump is connected to the electrical panel through a 25 amp circuit breaker, to protect the pump circuit.

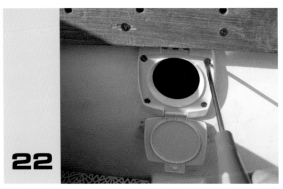

22

▲ A new manual bilge pump is installed in the same place as the old one – easily accessible in the cockpit, even when you are steering.

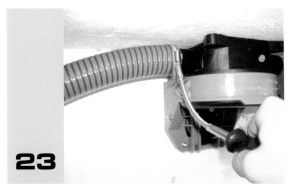

23

▲ The manual pump is heavily built and has a large capacity, at least for as long as the crew stay. The discharge fitting was installed on the opposite side of the hull from the electrically powered pump discharges.

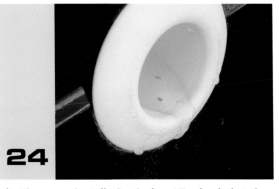

24

▲ The pump installation is done! To check that they worked, I performed one last test with a couple of buckets of water.

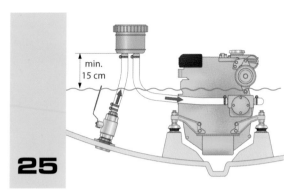

25

▲ Time for the filters! The base of the sea water strainer should be at least 15 cm/6 inches above the waterline. I put mine 30 cm above the waterline.

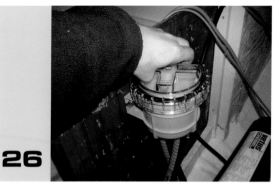

26

▲ The new water strainer. I bought an oversized Vetus strainer with a transparent plastic lid and it's carefully considered location, so that it would be easy to see when the filter screen needs to be emptied and cleaned.

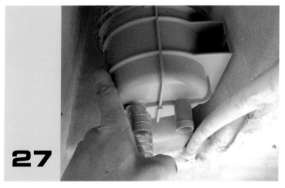

27

▲ I placed the bilge water filter/separator as high up as possible. This device will prevent oil and other contaminants from escaping into the sea with the bilge water.

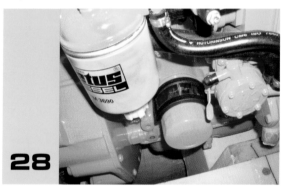

28

▲ The engine oil filter has a powerful magnet that attracts metal particles smaller than those that the filter element (10 micron) can trap.

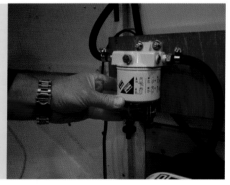

29

▲ A pre-filter (10 micron) takes care of particles and water at the first stage of the route from the tank to the engine. It can process 57 litres of fuel per hour; a lot more than *Roobarb*'s new engine demands.

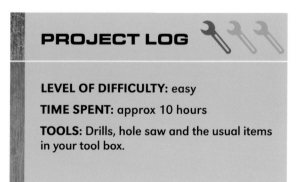

PROJECT LOG

LEVEL OF DIFFICULTY: easy

TIME SPENT: approx 10 hours

TOOLS: Drills, hole saw and the usual items in your tool box.

The pumps aboard *Roobarb*

Most pumps claim to have impressive pumping ability; in some cases thousand of litres or gallons per hour, but it's important to understand that this stated capacity is almost always given for no lift or head and zero back pressure. Even on my little boat *Roobarb*, the lift is more than 2 m/6 feet, resulting in the actual volume of water pumped out being only a fraction of the stated capacity. This is further reduced by bends in the hose, check valves, bilge water filters (strum boxes), etc.

It's hard to predict exactly how much water a pump will move once installed – many factors take effect including the quality of the installation.

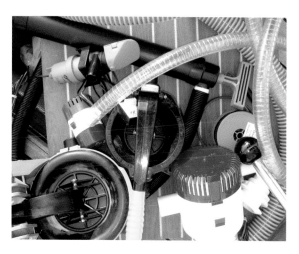

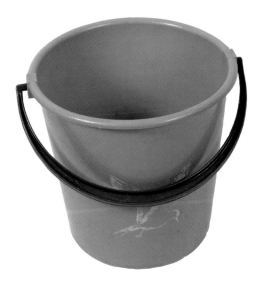

The Bucket, £2/$4. A frightened crew member with a bucket in hand, is one of the oldest, least expensive and most effective bilge pumping systems ever invented. There are several buckets on board Roobarb.

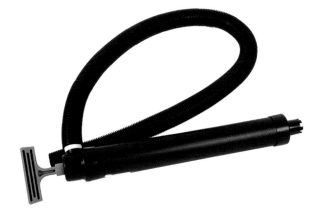

This hand pump (£40/$65) works by pulling a piston through a cylinder, which is fitted with a one-way valve at the water intake. It's simple and easy to use to suck up small quantities of water. The plastic pipe did not fit well on the one I bought, and I had to tape it in place. The hand pump is very light and easy to move to pockets and puddles that don't drain to the bilge.

Boat talk

Bilge water is dirty water that collects in the lowest part of the hull of a ship or boat. It is usually the result of below-the-waterline leaks, seas and spray breaking over the boat, rain and condensation. The bilge, where this water collects, is often difficult to access, making it hard to remove the water unless fixed pumps are installed at the lowest points or in sumps.

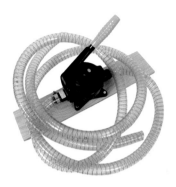

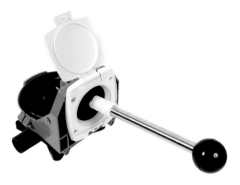

Portable diaphragm pump, £45/$60.

I bolted this inexpensive pump to a plywood base that I stand on when pumping, to stabilize the pump. The permanently attached hoses, with a combined length of 5 m/16 feet can reach from the front of the bilge to the galley sink.

Large diaphragm pump, £90/$120.

I replaced the old manual bilge pump. The old pump was a Whale Gusher Mk 8, but I could not find a ready supply of spares for it. So I installed a newer 'Gusher Titan' which is the updated version of the pump from the Whale company. The pump was installed on the bridge deck in the same place as the old pump and is worked from the cockpit by the helmsman, who can reach both the tiller and the pump handle. A little filler in the old bolt holes and a drill for the new holes were all that was needed to complete the upgrade.

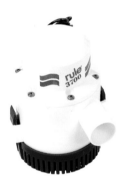

The high capacity emergency pump, approx £130/$190.

The large emergency bilge pump, like the small pump, is centrifugal. I mounted it on a stainless steel carrier, slightly more than 10 cm/4 inches above the lowest part of the bilge. It is turned on manually and used when there is more water than the little pump can handle. The emergency pump has a capacity of 230 litre/60 US gallons per minute and uses 15.5 amps of electrical current at 12 volts, so it needs plenty of battery power, and battery charging capacity, to keep going for very long. The maximum height of delivery or head is 6 metres or 18 feet, but that much lift will, of course, drastically reduce the flow rate or capacity.

If the emergency pump, with a nominal capacity of almost 14,000 litres/3,700 US gallons per hour is still not enough, I can shut a seacock and disconnect a hose so that the engine cooling system draws raw water from the flooded bilge. Not a happy thought, but you've got to have a plan, and a back-up plan, for emergencies at sea.

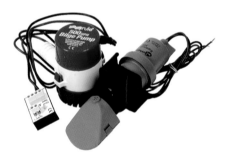

Small submersible pump, approx £30/$45.

By far the most widely used bilge pumps on recreational boats, these are not self-priming and must be submerged to pump, although they can run dry without damage. Roobarb's new bilge pump had a nominal capacity of 32 litres/ 8.5 US gallons per minute at zero lift (ie with no hose attached). I tested it with a lift of 2 m/6 feet to discover that in that situation, it could only pump a fraction of its nominal capacity. I had expected the capacity to be lower than the stated nominal flow rate, both because of the height of the required lift from the bilge to the discharge fitting and because I had installed an extra bilge water filter or strum box on the pump intake port. The diameter of the pump was only 60 mm/2 inches, a wider pump would not have fitted in the narrow space at the bottom of the bilge in Roobarb.

FOCUS FUEL FILTERS

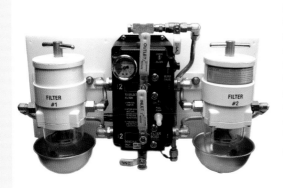

Fuel management systems are available for recreational boats, such as this Filter-Boss unit from KTI Systems. It consists of a fuel pump, dual Racor filters (2, 10 or 30 micron) and a warning mechanism that sounds an alarm if there is a reduction in the flow of diesel, requiring a filter change. The Filter-Boss pump can also be used to bleed air from the fuel system, as a fuel pump to move diesel from the tank to the engine or as part of an onboard fuel polishing system.

The Filter-Boss package shown retails for about £1,200/$1,600.

Diesel engines are very reliable, provided their supply of fuel is not contaminated by dirt, organic sludge or water, all of which will block filters and damage pumps and injection nozzles. In addition, leaks can couse problems in engines by allowing air into the fuel system.

Fuel filter elements come in different gradations of weave and tension (filtering ability), so that they can trap dirt particles of different sizes and can, in some cases, stop water. Filter elements are available in particle filtering ability from 45 microns to less than 1 micron, with 10 and 30 microns being the most common grades in recreational marine applications. A one micron particle has a diameter of one millionth of a metre.

Almost all diesel engines have an attached secondary filter, graded at ten microns, to trap any small particles that have passed through the primary fuel filter/water separator installed in the fuel hose between the tank and the engine.

Formula for calculating suitable capacity for the primary (coarse) filter:

Engine output in horsepower (hp) x 0.68 = capacity in litre per hour.

Example: 25 hp x 0.68 = 17 litres (4.5 US gallons) per hour.

INSTALLATION OF DOUBLE FILTERS

A good setup is to have dual filter canisters, mounted parallel in one assembly, so that when the first element is blocked or waterlogged, you can simply turn a valve to switch to the other canister without stopping the engine.

These multiple canister filter assemblies are fitted with three-way valves so that the new canister can come on line before the fouled canister is shut off. One of these assemblies may be ideal if you sail in heavy weather and big seas or in locations where an engine shutdown could lead to a disaster. If you're at sea in rough conditions, with the boat being thrown around, it can be very difficult, even nauseating, to change the element on a single canister filter and then bleed the fuel system before you can get going again. Some advice: don't be cheap and undersize the filter – it's an inexpensive component that protects your very expensive engine. At any price it's an insurance bargain, engine insurance and life insurance.

Don't put alcohol-based water absorbers in your fuel tank – they allow suspended water in the fuel to bypass the separator component of the fuel filter, with the potential to seriously damage your engine.

07
SOUND, AIR, POWER AND FIRE

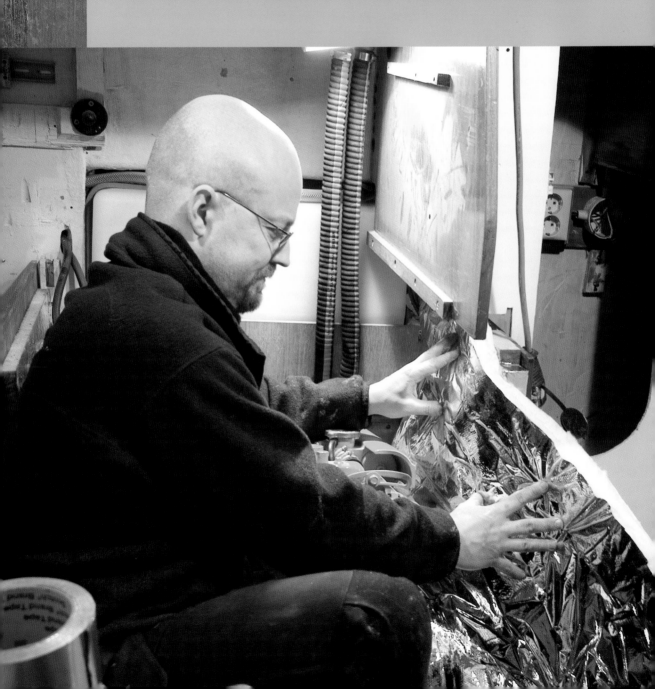

>> QUIET(ER) AT LAST

A pleasant side effect of changing the engine was a reduction in noise – the new engine is quieter than the old one. In addition, I installed sound-deadening materials around the engine space, which made things even quieter. And who doesn't enjoy peace and quiet on a boat?

Fire protection and exhaust systems are also discussed in this chapter, as we approach the end of the repower project.

When I was running the old engine, there was so much noise that I had to shut the companionway hatch before I could hear myself talk in the cockpit. The racket came from the shaking and vibration of the old horizontal single-cylinder Yanmar YSE12, and the vibration from it that passed into the hull and caused everything else to shake, rattle (and roll).

The new, three-cylinder engine with its flexible mounts, does not suffer from these problems, and the space under the cockpit that used to amplify the engine noise is now lined with acoustic material and filled with the big (215 litre) fuel tank.

New sound insulation panels, made mostly of foamed plastic, and micro-fibre padding have reduced the noise, although some still gets out of the engine space.

CHOICE OF SOUND INSULATION MATERIALS

The old foamed-plastic acoustic material had soaked up a lot of dirt and soot in its years of service. The new, smaller engine afforded more room for insulation but was also intrinsically quieter. When airborne sound needs to be reduced, insulating material must have an absorption function, so that the sound waves go into the material and are dissipated. Insulating materials must have open, porous and soft surfaces that don't reflect sound waves.

An effective noise-reduction programme reduces both structural and airborne vibration and noise. Only a small fraction of the engine noise in a boat is transferred directly from the engine to the air, most perceived noise comes from vibration transmitted through the hull to every other part, component and contents of the boat. Damping this structural vibration is essential but difficult.

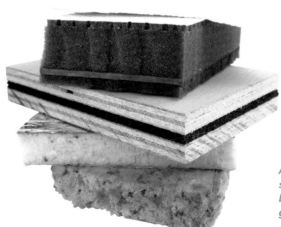

A lot of materials were considered for the sound proofing for the new engine. At the bottom is the old insulation that were old and gritty. The other will be covered on page 114.

10 tips for a quieter engine

1. Select the softest engine mounts that will work with your engine.
2. Make sure that the engine-gearbox assembly and the shaft are aligned, with an in-water check if alignment was performed on the dry.
3. A CV joint or flexible coupling reduces vibration.
4. Install an additional muffler in the exhaust system.
5. Acoustically line empty spaces that could act as amplifiers.
6. Use bitumen mats in or under foam sound insulation.
7. For effective sound insulation, use the thickest foamed plastic panelling that will fit the space.
8. Seal all cracks and openings in the engine enclosure, to stop airborne noise.
9. Different insulating materials absorb or block different types of noise.
10. Providing it's spiral reinforced to prevent kinking, flexible (soft and pliable) exhaust hose is better than rigid hose.

I chose a simple approach, buying inexpensive 20 mm/¾" inch foamed polyester panels. These became the first layer of acoustic material around the engine space. The price was less than £10/$16 for a 100 x 50 cm/3' 4" x 1' 8" piece. These panels were then supplemented with more modern materials; Thinsulate is best known as an insulation layer in outdoor clothing and ski gloves, but it can also act as an efficient sound insulation blanket in engine rooms. Its layer of micro fibre fabric protected on both sides by a foil are able to absorb the energy in sound waves very well.

What the boat lacks in effective sound insulation is bitumen-based padding – a mat of heavy and dense material that reduces vibration on any surface to which it is glued (or painted). I can always buy some of

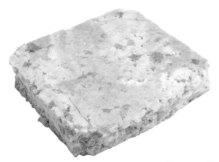

The 30-year-old sound proofing was dirty and not very effective. It was removed and two layers of new insulation were installed.

this later, if the noise level needs to be further reduced, even if it means tearing out some of the newly installed foamed plastic. Valve noise transmitted back through the combustion air intake of the engine was the hardest to reduce. You can read more about air supply later in this chapter. Acoustically insulating an engine space is not a technically complex matter, but the inaccessibility and irregular shape of the space can make installing acoustic materials a difficult and time consuming task.

AIR SUPPLY

A 25 hp internal combustion engine consumes about 113 cubic meters/3,990 cubic feet of air per hour. That's a lot of air and the engine spaces of many boats with inboard engines are not adequately ventilated to provide that air, resulting in reduced power and the black smoke that comes from incomplete combustion of diesel fuel. Another effect of inadequate ventilation is that the engine space becomes too hot, leading to reduced power and increased fuel consumption.

The rule of thumb is that a compression ignition (diesel) internal combustion engine consumes 6.1 cubic meters/215 cubic feet of air to produce one kilowatt of power, or 4.5 cubic meter/159 cubic feet of air to produce one horse power. By weight, the combustion of a kilogram of diesel requires 16 kg of air and one pound of diesel requires 16 pounds of air.

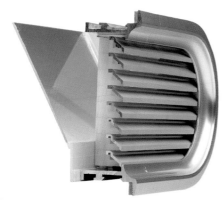

A louvered air suction vent from Vetus with a simple water baffle. This is an engine combustion air intake. I chose a different way to supply Roobarb's engine air, from the inside of the boat; through the bilge.

Before starting this installation I needed to know how much air the new engine would need, how much vent area would be required to provide that air and how I should design and position the air intake to minimize noise.

The theoretical open surface area of the intake vent required for my new engine was one square decimetre (10 x 10 cm) or 15.5 square inches. The first plan was to put a louvered vent somewhere low down in the cockpit, directly above the engine, but a long-distance sailor must be prepared for having the boat pooped by a following sea, and a cockpit full of water. To avoid getting water into the air vent, I followed the advice of my expert aid to let the engine get its air from the bilge and through less purpose-made openings into the engine room. To keep the engine space cool, there must also be air outlets to facilitate cross-flow of air. However, don't attempt to put extractor fans in the engine room, the suction power of the engine's air intake will overpower them, resulting in overheating and damage to the fans.

In conflict with ventilation requirement, if the engine space is not air-tight you may find that an automatic fire extinguisher does not function properly. You can read more about my trials and tribulations with fire extinguishers and an unsealed engine room on the next page.

In addition to all of these issues, a dedicated engine air intake is also the most difficult noise source to quieten.

In conclusion, drawing the combustion air from inside the boat may not have been the ideal solution, but it was a necessary compromise to give me what I wanted on *Roobarb*, because my top priority was keeping water out of the engine space in the event of a flooded cockpit or a knock-down. Second among my concerns was reducing the noise level in the cockpit and saloon, closely followed by having means of a fixed fire extinguisher in the engine room.

ELECTRICAL SYSTEM

The new power cables for the starter of the new engine were quite short, from the red positive terminal of the starting battery to the starter solenoid, and from the black negative terminal of the battery to an earth/ground negative stud on the engine.

On *Roobarb*, the negative stud side was an engine tie-down bolt, with the area around the bolt hole stripped of paint to ensure good electrical contact. This location was recommended by the engine dealer after reviewing all the possible negative earth/ground locations.

Different engines and installations may require different negative earth/ground locations at which to connect the black power cable from the starting battery, but wherever you make this connection on the engine, it must be a substantial stud providing excellent electrical conductivity to the engine block and all of the electrical components that use the their mounting on the engine to make the negative side of a circuit. If in doubt about this, ask the engine dealer for advice, and be aware that if you use a bolt on an aluminium engine leg (as fitted to my new engine), the connection may not work as well as a direct connection to a cast iron engine block.

I decided not to earth/ground all the components in the drive train, such as the propeller shaft and shaft seal housing, by connecting them to each other and back to the engine block (often called bonding), but be aware that there are differing opinions on this and everything else related to earthing/grounding/bonding the underwater metal parts of a boat. It's wise to study the issue, seek advice from experienced marine technicians, and for a couple of years carefully monitor the system you install to check for corrosion at each connection and component, until you're sure that the way you've rigged it is working.

The first approach I considered was to have had a two kilo carbon dioxide extinguisher, modified a little so that the gas canister could be outside engine enclosure. The nozzle was to have a short hose running through the bulkhead to the top of the engine space for maximum effectiveness. There would be a manual pull handle in the cockpit to avoid the need to find and squeeze the extinguisher handle in a smoke-filled cabin. What worried me about this arrangement was that I thought that the carbon dioxide released by the extinguisher could replace the air in the interior of the boat, with the risk of asphyxiation for anyone sleeping or trapped below, a particular concern with small children.

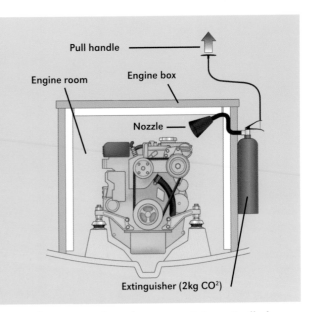

Pull handle

Engine room

Engine box

Nozzle

Extinguisher (2kg CO²)

An early sketch of a simple and inexpensive fire suppression system, based on a remotely controlled carbon dioxide extinguisher containing 2 kg/4.4 pounds of gas. This idea was quickly abandoned.

On the other side, the fill fittings of the fuel tanks are earthed/grounded, but not the tanks themselves as they are plastic. Metal tanks should always be earthed/grounded.

All other electrical circuits and functions were integrated with the engine wiring by pre-ended wiring harnesses/looms that were ready to attach to the engine control panel mounted in a cockpit bulkhead. All of the wires in the looms/harnesses came connected to multi-point plugs, so all I had to do was push them together. That was it – plug and play!

While the engine was out of *Roobarb*, and access temporarily improved, I took the opportunity to replace several parts of the general wiring system, but as that work was not directly related to the repower project, I'm not going to cover it in this book.

FIRE PROTECTION

A fire at sea is something to be avoided at all costs. According to the US Coast Guard's statistics, the most common cause (90%) of fires in engine rooms is leaking fuel. Dried-out fuel hoses crack and diesel fuel, (that can become volatile at around 50°C/120°F) touches the hot engine, evaporates, and if there is a source of ignition, such as an electrical spark, it catches fire.

Petrol/gasoline is much more flammable than diesel and vaporizes easily, which makes filling up more potentially dangerous. I suggest filling up while your family are away from the boat (send them for ice cream, etc) and be sure to run the bilge blowing fans for at least five minutes before starting any gasoline engine.

An engine room must be kept clean, with no oil or dirt to fuel a fire. A common cause of fire is a spark or short-circuit in the electrical system. Before this project, I had two 2 kg/4 pound dry powder fire extinguishers on board, one next to the companionway stairs and easily reached from the cockpit, the other in a cockpit locker.

The downside of dry powder extinguishers is that they make an awful mess, requiring a lot of clean-up, which can take weeks. For the engine room on a boat, gas extinguishers (for example FE200, carbon dioxide (CO_2) or water mist) are better.

When checking the alternatives, I considered several options, but the over-riding criteria was maximum safety for the crew at a price I could afford, and from a system requiring minimal maintenance. The basic idea was to keep things as simple as possible, and I changed direction several times while searching for the best fire prevention solution for *Roobarb*.

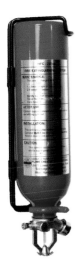

A fixed extinguisher with an automatic release is a safe but expensive fire suppression system for a small recreational boat.

A fixed automatic extinguishing system was attractive but the price and complexity of the systems I investigated made me a bit hesitant.

On such a small boat, just 8 mm/26 feet overall, I'm never far away from any of the extinguishers on board. On a bigger boat, with an engine room that's hard to reach quickly from the cockpit, an automatic extinguisher system, combined with heat and smoke detectors, is the only way to go because by the time you can smell a fire or see smoke, the fire may be too large to put out.

FIXED EXTINGUISHER

An automatic extinguisher usually incorporates a fusible link that melts at approx. 80° C/176° F, releasing the extinguishing substance into the protected space. Such an extinguisher may also have some other type of activating sensor, but the

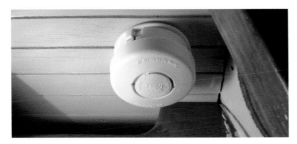

An inexpensive optical fire alarm sounds when there is smoke in the cabin, but don't place it too close to the stove – at least not if you burn food as often as I do...

advantage of a fusible link is that it doesn't require a power source or electrical connection, and works when everything else on the boat is turned off or out of action.

Something to think about when installing a fixed gas extinguisher is that the engine room must be air tight for the extinguisher is to work properly. Openings under the engine and into the bilge must be sealed, so that the heavier-than-air extinguishing gas doesn't drain away before the fire is out. Initially I had intended to do this with the same foamed-plastic acoustic panels that I had used to line the rest of the engine space. Instead of gluing the panels into place, I made them a press fit, in the hope that they could be easily removed for engine maintenance.

An automatic extinguisher system should include an automatic engine cut-off switch that also controls the bilge blowers so that the extinguishing gas or vapor is not extracted by the engine air intake or the bilge blower fans. On a boat with an electric fuel pump and shut-off valve between the fuel tank and the engine, those should also be connected to the extinguisher control circuits and automatically turned off in the event of a fire.

For maximum fire suppression, automatic dampers would be installed on the air intake vents to the engine space, but so far at least, I've only heard of that on large vessels. If you can find a way to shut the intake vents on your boat, in the event of a fire, set it up. In the end I settled for a powder extinguisher and a woven fibreglass fire blanket, stowed in the galley, as the fire suppression system on *Roobarb*.

I installed a Fire Port fitting in the top of the engine enclosure, so that in the event of an engine room fire, it will be possible to insert the nozzle of the powder extinguisher into the engine space without increasing the air supply to the fire by opening an access panel or hatch. A very important added benefit of the Fire Port is that it eliminates the possibility of the fire blowing back and engulfing you when you open an access panel or hatch to the burning engine space.

EXHAUST SYSTEM

In a 'wet' exhaust system, the raw water discharged from the engine cooling system is injected into the hot exhaust gas (up to 600° C or 1,100° F) in a mixing elbow bolted to the end of the engine exhaust manifold. This reduces the temperature of the exhaust gas to around 45°C/113°F, and also drastically reduces the volume and pressure of the gas (Boyle's Law). This reduction of temperature, volume and pressure alone greatly reduces the noise of the exhaust.

The mixing elbow is a weak point in the wet exhaust system, and is invariably the first component to wear out, as the result of constant exposure to a very corrosive mix of hot gases and salt water. On some engines this happens after only a few years. The solution may be to change to a stainless steel elbow but that costs more than bronze and is less able to handle vibration. The mixing elbows used by Vetus and Yanmar are made of bronze, and after-market stainless steel mixing elbows are available for many engines including the old Volvo Penta units.

At first, I thought I might be able to keep some of the existing exhaust system components, but I soon realized that they were worn out and also not the required sizes for the new engine. There are adaptor hose fittings to go from one dimension to another but the hoses had dried out and needed changing anyway.

On a cruise a couple of years ago with the old engine, black smoke filled the boat as a result of the mixing elbow snapping off where it had rusted through. With twenty miles still to go, we drifted for a while as I made a stop-gap repair by wrapping the broken elbow with leather, bound in place with steel wire and hose clamps. I'm embarrassed to admit that my stop-gap measure stayed in place till the end of that summer (I know – Physician, heal thyself!).

A new bronze mixing elbow replaced the old cast iron component, even though the connection adaptor to the outlet of the exhaust manifold was still easily-corroded cast iron.

The simplest possible wet exhaust system would be a hose from the engine to a transom exhaust outlet preferably run through a gooseneck bend. However, a properly designed system will include a water lock to capture water running back from the top of the gooseneck towards the engine on shut down. The gooseneck prevents a following sea flooding the exhaust hose and engine, the water lock captures backflow, and they are both essential elements of a wet exhaust system.

The main problem I encountered when planning the new exhaust system for *Roobarb* was that there was no good place to put the water lock, which needed to be lower than the mixing elbow. I got it is as low as I could, so that it was sitting over the extended shaft log, supported by hangers attached to the large fuel tank. All boats are different and there are many different water locks to meet the exhaust system requirements of a particular boat.

If the water-lock products of one manufacturer

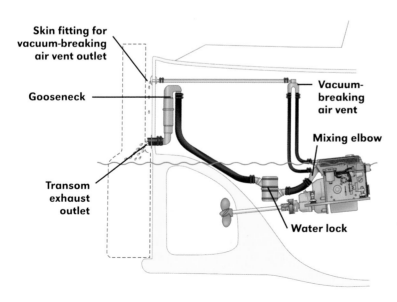

Skin fitting for vacuum-breaking air vent outlet

Gooseneck

Vacuum-breaking air vent

Mixing elbow

Transom exhaust outlet

Water lock

A sketch of how the exhaust system on **Roobarb** *is designed. It's fairly similar to a standard installation, with a water lock and gooseneck. The vacuum-breaking air vent valve has an overflow at the transom, providing a clear and simple signal that the raw water side of the cooling system is working properly. Warning! an improperly designed and sized wet exhaust system, or a missing or improperly located vacum-braking air vent, can cause your new engine to be damaged beyond repair at the first start up or shut down. The damage is not covered by the engine waranty, so if you are not sure about any of this, consult an expert.*

don't solve the exhaust system problems on your boat, try a different manufacturer. In a very cramped engine space with a deep bilge it may even be possible to position the water-lock under the engine, as has been done on quite a few boats.

As mentioned, I attached a Vetus plastic gooseneck fitting to the transom exhaust outlet with a short length of exhaust hose. This gooseneck will prevent a wave that surges over the stern from filling the exhaust system and flooding the engine. A rubber flap in the transom exhaust fitting provides some additional protection, as it closes and acts as a one-way valve when submerged.

A transom exhaust fitting should be at least 5cm/2 inches above the surface of the water, although more is better. Locating the exhaust outlet on the centre of the transom will prevent the exhaust outlet from being submerged when the boat is heeled, rail down in a blow. The engine cooling system and exhaust system meet at the mixing elbow, providing another, more insidious, route for water to get into the engine, so the water hose feeding the mixing elbow must be fitted with an air vent to prevent back-flooding and siphonage.

VACUUM-BREAKING AIR VENT

A vacuum-breaking air vent is necessary if the engine is partly or completely installed below the waterline, as is the case on most sailing boats. This air-vent stops the siphon effect when the engine is turned off and the water in the hose above the mixing elbow flows down through the elbow and into the water lock. If that goes on for just a few minutes, the water lock will fill up, the water will rise up to the mixing elbow and flow from there along the exhaust manifold and into the engine through any open valve. This is a very common cause of engine damage and destruction, can happen to a brand new engine and is not covered by the manufacturer's warranty – it's an installation mistake. A vacuum breaking air-vent should be mounted as high as possible, at least 40 cm above the water surface, and once again, near the centreline so that it is not flooded when the boat is heeled, rail down or pooped by a following sea. Some vacuum valves (including some from Volvo Penta) can leak a bit when starting up and turning off the engine, before the internal valve closes. A small

metal bowl will catch this water, but it's a good idea to make sure that nothing that can be damaged by water that is placed under the air vent device.

Some airvents do not have a valve at all, but instead a small hose connected to a breather fitting mounted high on the topsides. The breather fitting will spurt a little water whenever the engine is running, and if that water flow stops, it's a sure sign that the raw water supply to the engine has stopped, either from a blockage, or more likely, a failed impeller in the raw water pump of the engine. This works as a useful tell-tale, and indicates an immediate engine shut down, before the exhaust system is heat damaged, which will happen before the engine temperature rises significantly.

Annual maintenance is required for any air vent with a valve, as salt will build up on the spring or joker valve, requiring thorough cleaning, and probably replacement of the moving parts of the valve.

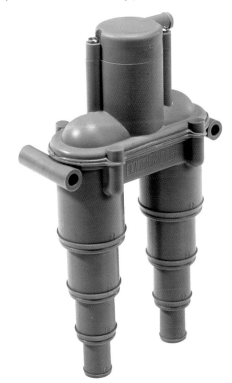

A simple type of vacuum-breaking air vent, with no valve to get stuck and a tell-tale overboard water flow that shows when the raw water side of the cooling system is working properly.

>> STEP-BY-STEP

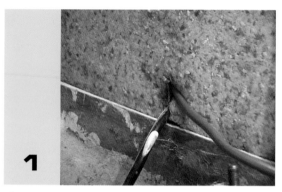

▲ First project out is sound proofing. The thirty-year-old sound insulation had seen better days.

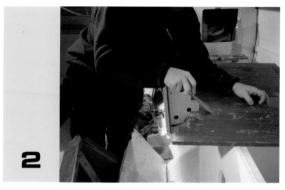

▲ The old material was scraped and ground from the inside of the engine box. Unfortunately, the glue was still very well attached.

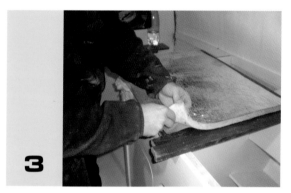

▲ All flat surfaces were covered with inexpensive plastic foam insulation, supplied in self-adhesive panels.

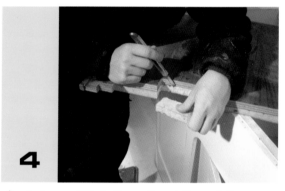

▲ A sharp utility knife easily cut through the material. I had to cut and fit to match the new insulation to the irregular shape of the engine box or enclosure.

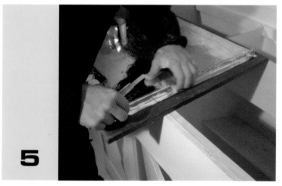

▲ All joints and edges were covered in self-adhesive aluminium tape, to keep dirt and oil fumes away from the foamed plastic.

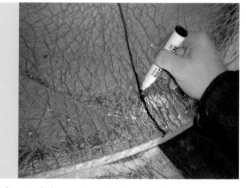

▲ The front of the engine box had an irregular shape and required me to cut several small pieces, which went together like a jigsaw puzzle.

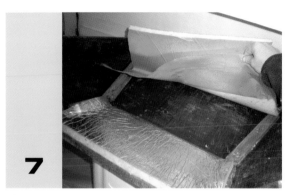

▲ It was quite difficult to fit the uneven bits together but the self-adhesive insulation made it easier to end up with a neat job.

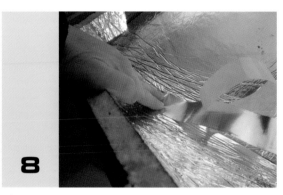

▲ Even the joints between the sections are taped together to create a closed surface that will not let dirt in or sound out.

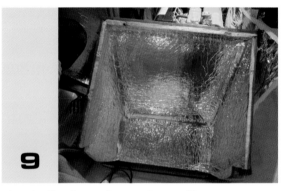

▲ The first layer of acoustic panelling was complete, except for taping the exposed edges of the foam.

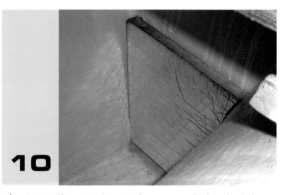

▲ A set of acoustic panels was made for the bilge. These are removable if it becomes apparent that the engine is not getting enough air for complete combustion.

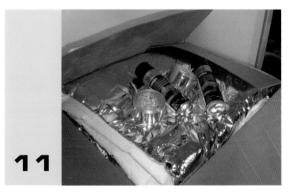

▲ I chose to have a second layer of sound proofing, this time made of Thinsulate fabric. It is applied to the engine box with the recommended spray adhesive and aluminium tape, which all were included in the box.

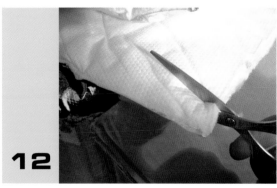

▲ The Thinsulate acoustic padding consists of insulating microfibre, protected from dirt by a layer of aluminium foil. The padding is easy to shape with a standard pair of scissors.

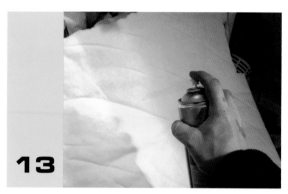

13

▲ The padding can be secured with stainless steel staples or with spray adhesive which seemed easier to me. I applied the adhesive to the back of the padding...

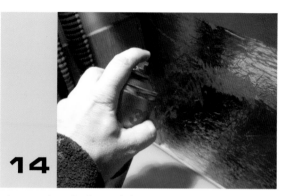

14

▲ ...and to the face of the engine box panels, to which it was being attached. This is contact adhesive so it grabs immediately – you've got to get it in the right place on the first attempt.

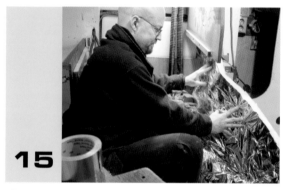

15

▲ The acoustic padding is as soft as an eiderdown bedcover and very easy to handle and install.

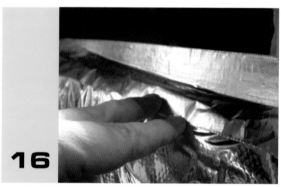

16

▲ The edges of the insulation were sealed with aluminium tape, which was a little tricky and tore if I didn't pay close attention.

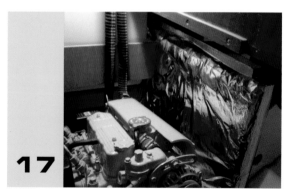

17

▲ I was pleased with the results of my labour, and made sure that the insulation was not touching any moving parts.

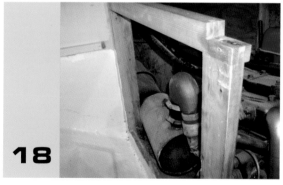

18

▲ The next project was the exhaust system and I'd hoped that I'd be able to re-use the old one, but the hoses didn't fit the new engine, and everything was more or less worn out.

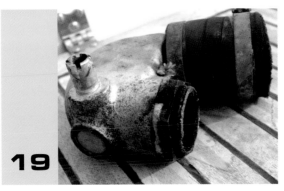

19

▲ The old cast iron mixing elbow to the old engine had cracked during a week-end of sailing, a couple of years ago, and had been replaced with a bronze elbow. This is a common problem. I scrapped everything.

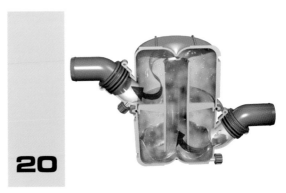

20

▲ The core component of the new exhaust system is a modern water-lock, with upper and lower sections that rotate relative to each other, and swiveling intake and discharge fittings. This also functions as a very effective silencer/muffler.

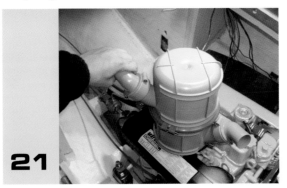

21

▲ With its rotating body and swiveling connections, this water-lock will work in the most awkward and tight situations.

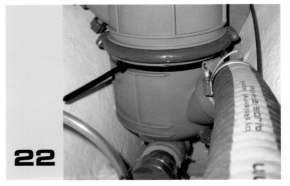

22

▲ The water-lock was held in place by plastic hangers, attached to the main fuel tank support. The water-lock also gained some additional support from the shaft log.

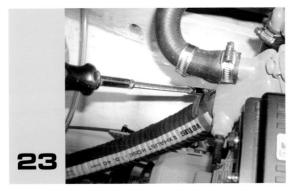

23

▲ The exhaust hose was attached to the exhaust elbow with double, marine-grade, hose clamps.

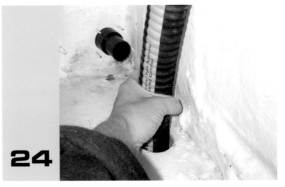

24

▲ In completing the exhaust installation, I drilled new holes in the interior to make the hose run as straight as possible.

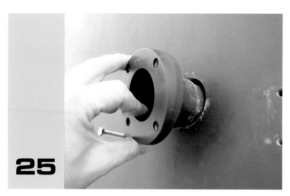

25

▲ The exhaust outlet was a new plastic transom fitting, bedded in sealant and bolted into place.

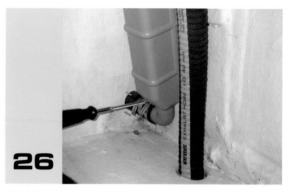

26

▲ The gooseneck will prevent large waves from flooding the exhaust system and engine. A short length of exhaust hose connected the gooseneck to the transom exhaust fitting.

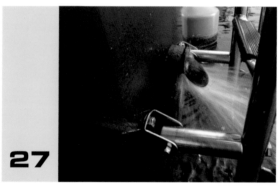

27

▲ The transom exhaust fitting has a rubber flap that closes when submerged, providing additional protection against waves surging over the stern and flooding the exhaust system and engine.

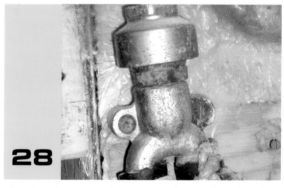

28

▲ For the next project I wanted to replace the old vacuam-breaking air vent as it had definately seen its best days. I did still work but leaked sometimes on the engine.

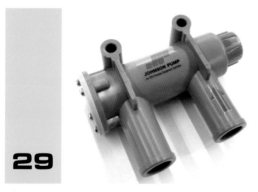

29

▲ An air vent is an important part of a wet exhaust system, preventing raw water from the engine cooling system being siphoned into the exhaust system and flooding the engine. Vacuum-breaking air vents are available from several manufacturers.

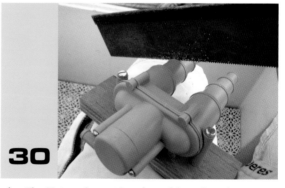

30

▲ The Vetus air vent is adaptable to four hose sizes, by simply cutting back the hose pillars so that the required diameter remains.

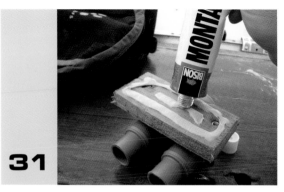

▲ The air vent was screwed to a wooden pad, which in turn was glued to the inner face of a cockpit bulkhead.

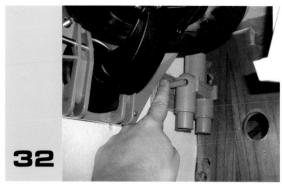

▲ The valve was placed as high as possible and as close as possible to the centre line of the boat. It was just over 80 cm/2′ 8″ inches above the waterline.

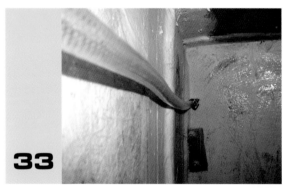

▲ The air vent hose was led to the transom. I had a few problems when dirt got into the hose and stopped the flow of water in the 1.5 m/5′ long hose that was later glued to the wall.

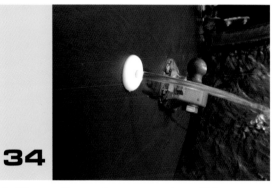

▲ The overflow at the transom shows if the vacuum-breaking air vent and the raw water side of the engine cooling system are working properly. Some air vents have air inlet valves and do not require an outlet hose.

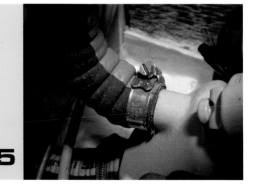

▲ The hose pillar on the mixing elbow was not a perfect fit to the hose and the clamp had to be forcefully tightened. The exhaust system was done!

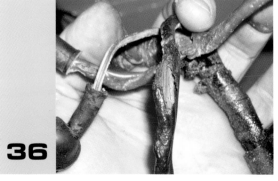

▲ The next step was to fit the electrical system. The old one had apparently short circuited and dubious repairs had been made with electrical tape. It was time for a change!

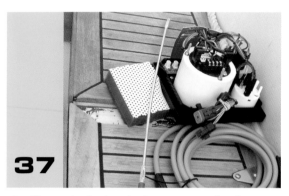

37

▲ The engine's electrical system was simple, consisting of two wiring looms/harnesses and an engine panel that I mounted in the cockpit.

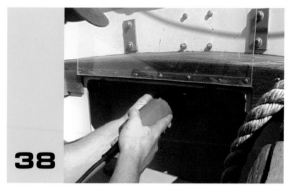

38

▲ Using the Fein oscillating saw, I managed to fit the engine instrument panel in a sheltered but somewhat awkward place at the back of the cockpit.

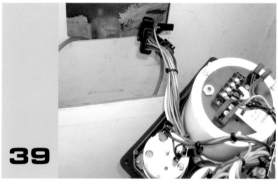

39

▲ Two wiring looms/harnesses go from the panel to the engine and are joined by quick connect plugs.

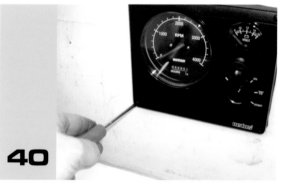

40

▲ The engine panel has a sturdy rubber gasket – it had to be watertight.

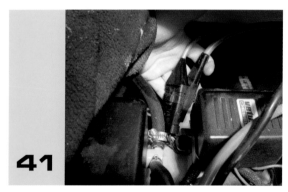

41

▲ The engine ends of the wiring looms/harnesses are connected to the engine. Done!

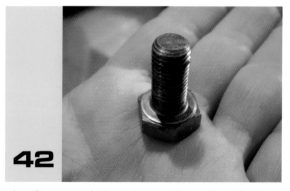

42

▲ After some deliberation on alternative solutions the negative side of the start battery bank was connected to the engine block, using this finely threaded bolt that originally was used to fix the engine to the transport cradle.

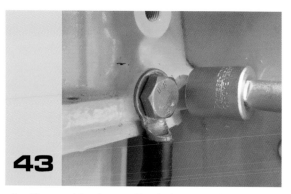

43

▲ The earthing/grounding bolt secured the black cable from the negative (minus) side of the battery to the engine block, providing earthing/grounding for all of the components of the engine electrical system.

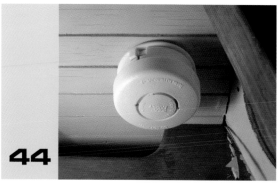

44

▲ The new fire protection system consists of several devices and components. The first of these is a simple fire alarm, attached to the cabin headlining above the engine enclosure.

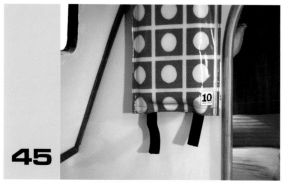

45

▲ The fire blanket hangs next to the galley and can be used for all small fires, not just frying pan flare-ups.

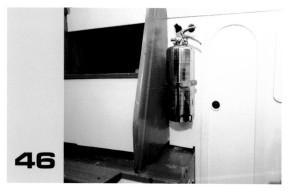

46

▲ One of the two dry-powder extinguishers was installed right next to the engine enclosure.

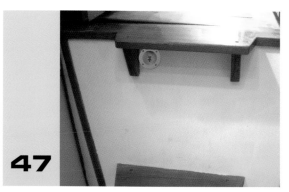

47

▲ The finishing touch is a 'Fire Port', in the top of the engine enclosure. The Fire Port has a split diaphragm, through which the nozzle of the adjacent fire extinguisher can be inserted, to put out an engine fire without opening the enclosure.

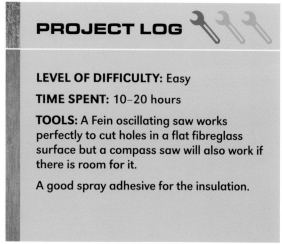

PROJECT LOG

LEVEL OF DIFFICULTY: Easy

TIME SPENT: 10–20 hours

TOOLS: A Fein oscillating saw works perfectly to cut holes in a flat fibreglass surface but a compass saw will also work if there is room for it.

A good spray adhesive for the insulation.

FOCUS WHAT'S IN A FIRE EXTINGUISHER?

There are different types of extinguisher for different types of fire:

POWDER EXTINGUISHER

Monoammonium Phosphate is the most common extinguishing agent in dry powder extinguishers and is suitable for use against Fire Classes A, B and C. Many other chemicals are used including Sodium Bicarbonate and Potassium Bicarbonate powder, (also known as 'Purple K'), each having different advantages and disadvantages, but all having the effect of coating the fuel and smothering the fire. Monoammonium Phosphate has the best extinguishing capability per kg/pound of the widely used powders, and is recommended for homes and boats. It is non-conductive and can be used on all common types of fire including electrical fires. The disadvantages of all powder extinguishing agents are that they reduce visibility and their residue is difficult to remove. Powder extinguishers should be shaken a few times each season.

FOAM EXTINGUISHERS

Most foam extinguishers contain water mixed with a soapy liquid that reduces the surface tension of the water, and also allows it to be aerated into a foam. This aqueous foam is an effective extinguisher for Type A and B fires of fibrous substances and burning liquids, although foam has limited effect on running liquids and gases. Water based foam is conductive and cannot be used against electrical fires.

The liquids in foam extinguishers freeze, so they cannot be left outside in sub-freezing temperatures.

WATER EXTINGUISHERS

Water is only suitable for extinguishing Type A fires in fibrous materials and has less effect than foam and powder. To prevent freezing, these extinguishers cannot be left outside in sub-freezing weather, and as water conducts electricity, they cannot be used against electrical fires. Water is

Fixed extinguishing systems

Until 1994, the inert gas, Halon (Bromotrifluoromethane), a very efficient extinguisher, was used worldwide in fire suppression systems. This gas prevents chain reactions in the fire and creates an anti-inflammatory atmosphere that suffocates the fire even at concentrations as low as a few percent of Halon in a Halon/air mixture. Unfortunately, the gas is bad for the environment and the ozone layer, and was prohibited for use in boats many years ago (1998 in Europe). Today there are replacement gases, such as FM-200 from Great Lakes Chemical or FE-227 from Du-Pont, that contain heptafluoropropane

An alternative to these is an extinguisher that injects water mist at high pressure into the location and effectively cools down the fire. A surprisingly small amount of this water mist is required to put out a fire and the mist does not damage electronic equipment.

The use of a powder extinguisher inserted through a fire port into the engine room can be a very efficient fire suppression method on a small boat, but unfortunately it is difficult to clean areas where powder has been used. It is also possible for powder to be sucked into the engine, resulting – at a minimum – in the need to completely dismantle it for cleaning. If you can summon the presence of mind while your boat is on fire, turn off the engine before using the dry powder extinguisher in the engine space. It's important to understand that even a small opening can provide fire-sustaining oxygen to an otherwise closed engine room.

In spite of the clean-up task, if you only have a powder extinguisher, you've got to use it quickly and without hesitation – the alternative is losing the boat.

also unsuitable for use against burning liquids such as fuel.

CARBON DIOXIDE EXTINGUISHERS

CO_2 extinguishers contain the gas Carbon Dioxide and are intended for use against fires in liquids and synthetic materials. Carbon dioxide is not very effective against fires in wood, paper or textiles and must be contained around the fire to prevent the gas flowing away and being replaced by combustion-supporting oxygen.

CO_2 is mainly used against fires in enclosed electrical equipment and engine spaces where it will not support combustion and leaves the scene of the fire with no residue or secondary damage.

INERT GASES

One of the most efficient extinguishers, the inert gas Halon has been prohibited for many years as it is extremely damaging to the ozone layer of the atmosphere. The replacements for Halon such as FE-227/FM200 (HFC-227ea, Heptafluoropropane) also work well and are available in fixed fire systems for boats. Research is under way to find new fire-suppression products and substances such as Aerosol and Novec may eventually become less expensive and thus more interesting to recreational boat owners.

CLASSIFICATION

One or more letters are marked on a fire extinguisher, to indicate the different types of fire for which the extinguisher is intended. Sometimes a number is added before the letter to indicate the effectiveness of the contents against particular type of fire. It could look something like '13A 89B C'. The higher the number, the higher the efficiency: Extinguishing effectiveness against Type A fires is rated from 5–55 and against Type B fires from 21-233, while extinguishers for Type C fires are not rated but are deemed by the manufacturers to be suitable for use against gas fires. Be aware that the letter classes for fires do not mean the same thing in every country, so when buying an extinguisher, read the label and instructions carefully.

TYPES OF FIRES

Fires of Class A and B are the most common in boats and in homes. **Class A** applies to fires in materials that burn with both flame and strong light. This includes most interior materials such as wood, sea charts, curtains and cushions. **Class B** applies to fires in liquids such as petrol or diesel. These burn with a flame but without strong light. In North America, Class B is also applied to fires of flammable gases. **Class C** applies to fires of flammable gases in Europe, Asia and Australasia, but also applies to electrical fires in North America. **Class D** applies to fires of combustible metals. **Class E** is discontinued in Europe, is not used in North America, but is still used in Asia and Australasia and applies to electric fires. Class F applies to fires of cooking oil or fat in Europe, Asia and Australasia, but is not used in North America. **Class K** applies to fires of cooking oil or fat in North America.

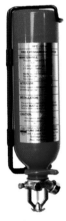

An automatic or remotely-controlled extinguisher eliminates the need to open the hatches to the engine space in the event of a fire.

Insulation materials

There are several types of sound insulation material than can be used on a recreational boat. Here are some of the most common:

FOAMED PLASTIC

The following are products that absorb airborne sound, some of them are composed of chunks of waste foam from other processes, pressed and glued into a single sheet or panel. Noise reduction occurs when sound waves penetrate the porous surface of the insulation, and then the sound's energy is absorbed in the soft and flexible foam interior. A thick layer of foamed plastic is more effective than a thin one.

Foamed plastic is often supplied with an outer layer of aluminium foil to protect the absorbent foam from spilled oil and airborne dirt. Foam panels are also available with fire-resistant surfaces and with self-adhesive backing that makes them easy to install on flat, clean surfaces. If the surfaces are not flat, foam panels can be screwed into place, using plate washers to minimize tearing the foil face.

HEAVY MAT

This absorbs structure-borne nose, using layers of bitumen (a petroleum product and an important component of asphalt) heat set into a pad of soundproofing, usually about 40 x 50 cm/16" x 20". The weight and mass of the mat reduces the ability of the surface to vibrate and transmit vibration and noise. These products weigh about 3 kilos per square metre/0.5 pounds per square foot depending on the thickness (usually around 2–3mm/1/8" thick) Bitumen based sound deadening mats are available in specialist car stores.

MICRO-FIBRE

This is to reduce airborne noise. Thinsulate is well known as thermal insulation in outdoor clothing and gloves, but also acts as a good acoustic insulation material. It's lightweight and water repellent (soaking up a mere 1% of its own weight in water). It's easy to cut to shape and can be glued or stapled into place. Thinsulate sound insulation only weighs 440 gram per square metre/1.5 ounces per square foot.

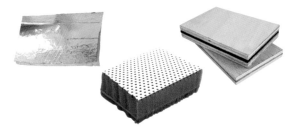

*Far left: Foamed plastic with aluminium foil facing.
Centre left: An effective sound proofing material consists of several layers, each good at absorbing different types of noise. This advanced sound board contains both bitumen and plastic foam, and costs approx £165 per square metre/$25 per square foot.
Left: Plywood with bitumen.*

Types of noise in boats

The Encyclopaedia defines sound as 'variations in pressure that spread out like waves. The original and narrow meaning was vibration in the air with a frequency between 20 and 20,000 Hz, and able to be heard by the human ear.'

On a boat, airborne sound is often high pitched and comes directly from the engine. It is reduced by absorbent materials such as soft, flexible foamed plastic. Structure-borne sound is that which is transmitted from the engine through the mounts and shaft and perceived as a dull, low frequency noise (an annoying sound). It can be reduced by covering large areas including the inside of the engine box and the hull with acoustic insulation or heavy padding that absorb or damp vibration. Vibrations transmitted through the boat's structure also cause other objects to vibrate, making more noise (very annoying sound) such as the rattling of coffee cups and glasses in the galley, although this is easily reduced by separating the vibrating items with bubble wrap, foam plastic, etc. Note that exhaust systems, steering cables and many other components make noise when they start vibrating, so it's important to tie back, clamp and stabilize everything possible.

Vacuum valves

Vacuum valves, or more properly, vacuum-breaking air vents, are intended to prevent a siphon developing in the hose from the engine cooling system to the mixing elbow of the wet exhaust system. When the engine is shut down, such a siphon can cause the exhaust system to fill with raw water, which then flows along the exhaust manifold, through any open valves and into the cylinders, with devastating results at the next attempt to start the engine.

One of these air vents, mounted at the high point of the raw water hose feeding the mixing elbow, breaks the siphon after the engine has stopped by allowing air into the hose, either by the opening of an air-intake valve (spring loaded or rubber joker type), or through a permanently open air hose connected to a breather fitting, high on the topsides of the hull. The traditional term for an unvalved vacuum breaker is a 'vented loop'.

The location of the vacuum-breaking air vent needs to be at least 40 cm/1' 4" above the waterline and on a sailboat as close as possible to the centreline so that the vent is still above the waterline when the boat is heeled rail down. Most of these vacuum valves are available with hose attachments from 12 to 25 mm/½ to 1 inch.

Some of the experts told me that it's not unusual for vacuum breakers to be left out by unqualified installers, often with disastrous consequences (always disastrous if the mixing elbow is below the waterline).

After installation, these devices need to be serviced annually to clear salt and other residue from the spring loaded valves, rubber joker valves and air intake tubes. If any of the small components is stuck or blocked, the anti-siphon function stops.

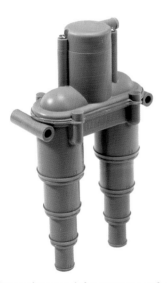

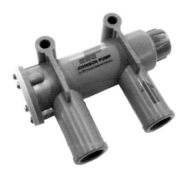

A new type of vacuum valve was engineered for Martec by the designer and sailor Lars Ljungberg after his engine was damaged when the vacuum breaker failed. It is also sold by Johnson Pump, and is available for five hose diameters (internal) from 12 to 25 mm/½ to 1 inch.

Vetus air vents (aka vacuum valves) are available in two versions, one valved and with no wet overflow, the other, which I chose for Roobarb, with an open overflow, a modern version of the traditional vented loop. The water flowing from this device is discharged through a transom breather fitting and is a useful indicator that the air vent and the raw water side of the engine cooling system are working properly – very simple, very clear. The overflow from an unvalved air vent can be run into the galley sink if you can't find a way to get it out on the topsides, although I don't much like the idea.

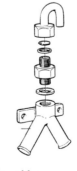

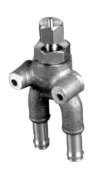

Traditional bronze vacuum valves are still available, from several manufacturers in a range of sizes (web search for details in your country).
To the left: Volvo Penta supplies vacuum-breaking bronze air vents and repair kits for them containing a spout cap, membrane and gasket.

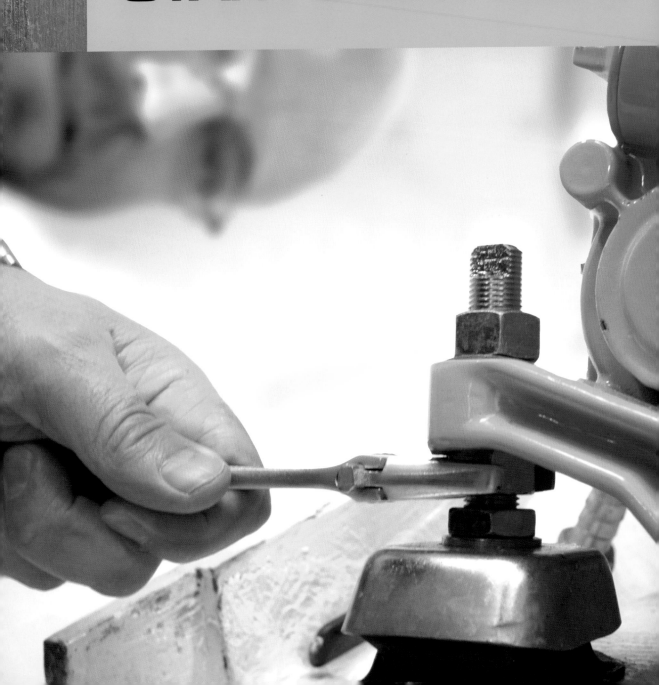

08

ALIGNMENT, TEST START & SEA TRIAL

HOW STRAIGHT IS STRAIGHT ENOUGH?

For a new engine and drive train to work well, it's essential that the engine is positioned on its bed so as to provide near perfect alignment between the output flange of the gearbox and the propeller shaft. I would now like to share some hard won insights into the process, cost and time involved in this repowering project.

It's easy to say that an engine connected to a rigid shaft must be positioned so that it is aligned with that shaft, but as with every boat job I tackled in this project for the first time, it seems is easier said than done.

Flexible shaft connections and CV-joints can make alignment less critical than it was before the advent of these devices, when the slightest inaccuracy resulted in excessive load and vibration on engine mounts, shaft seals and bearings, resulting in their premature failure.

I put considerable thought and effort into rebuilding the engine bed, mounting and aligning the engine and sound-proofing the engine enclosure to reduce the awful vibration and noise that shook the boat and filled the air whenever the old engine was running.

Like the borrowed jig, the face of the flexible shaft coupling was a great help in the alignment process, because it became possible to see with the naked eye if the coupling and the drive flange of the gearbox were parallel with each other, indicating good alignment. After reducing it to make room for the flexible coupling, *Roobarb*'s prop shaft is now very short. The length and diameter of the shaft must be checked in a repower project, as a long shaft may distort as a result of having to transmit more torque. A long shaft can also bend under its own weight and although a repower is not going to make an existing shaft any longer than it was, you may find that it's been sagging all along and needs support from an intermediate bearing.

Bo Linderholm of Alsten's Marine Tech, who helped and advised me throughout this project, said that it wasn't necessary to use feeler gauges to check for tenths of a millimetre in the parallel alignment of the gearbox drive flange and the flexible coupling face. Bo's experience has been that such small discrepancies are absorbed by the rubber core of the flexible coupling.

ENGINE MOUNTS

You can see how well you've succeeded in aligning the engine mounts with the engine bed, by using an inspection mirror if necessary, to look at them from different angles. To avoid uneven load distribution and stress, the mounts have to be straight in every direction, so that each takes an equal share of the engine's weight. Uneven loading causes vibration that can wear out the mounts and the prop shaft seals prematurely.

A simple way to check for even load distribution is to loosen the upper nuts of the engine mounts and then use a torque wrench to see how much force it takes to move each lower nut – if all of the lower nuts require equal force, the engine weight is evenly distributed.

Bo Linderholm pointed out that common sense should prevail, the torques are not going to be exactly the same, no matter how well you've done the installation. Not having his experience, I checked the torques on these load-carrying nuts several times to be sure I'd got it right.

It's also important to check that there is no twisting or side force on the rubber cores of the engine mounts when they are at rest, with the engine shut down. This can be done by loosening the hold down bolts, one mount at a time, and lifting that corner of the engine with a lever to take the load off the mount. If the mount shifts its position on the bed, it was side-loaded or twisted and needs to be repositioned.

Bo recommended using 8 mm bolts to hold the mounts down onto the engine bed, as they were slightly undersized to the holes in the base plates of the mounts, giving enough play to allow for small adjustments in the mount locations on the bed.

It's best to drill the bolt receiver holes in the engine beds with the engine in place and aligned, unless you have a very accurate jig. If the holes are just a few

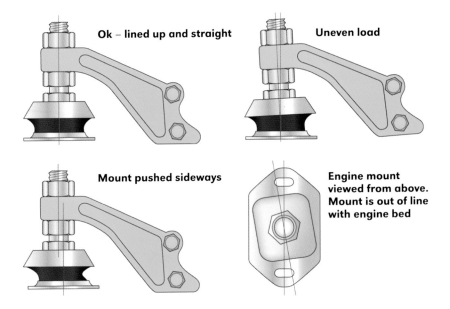

Ok – lined up and straight

Uneven load

Mount pushed sideways

Engine mount viewed from above. Mount is out of line with engine bed

The engine mounts have to be adjusted correctly in all directions so that there is no inner stress when they are at rest. Adjustments will be both vertical and horizontal and when you've made them, the threaded stud of the mount must be square to the receiver of the engine leg. Keep adjusting until you get it right!

millimetres out of place, the whole installation process can become much more difficult to complete well.

A good start is to check all of the critical dimensions on the drawings, the jig and the actual engine. If they're not the same, stop, think and resolve the differences before proceeding.

MORE ADJUSTMENTS

Most engine mounts can be adjusted vertically by raising or lowering the bearer nuts under the engine legs. It's often hard to get a new engine low enough in the boat to line up with the prop shaft – one boat owner told me that he'd cut holes in the hull and built fiberglass pockets, creating bumps on the exterior of the hull to to make low engine mount pads. Don't try this at home!

Do whatever it takes to the get engine bed right before going any further with the installation of a new engine. If you don't take the time to do this, there will be problems and unpleasant surprises throughout the installation process.

Final alignment of the engine-gearbox assembly and the propeller shaft must be performed when the boat is back in the water, as most hulls change shape between being blocked up ashore and floating. With a sailboat, the hull will also flex slightly as the standing rigging is tightened and tuned, so that also needs to be done before the final drive train alignment.

Although that's already more alignment work than any do-it-yourself boat owner ever dreamed necessary, two weeks after putting the boat back in the water it will all have to be checked and adjusted yet again, to compensate for the new engine mounts having compressed. In addition, the vibration of the new engine may loosen the nuts and bolts of the mounts, so these also need to be checked frequently during the first few months of operating the new engine.

KEEP AN EYE ON IT

Six months after the installation, with the boat back ashore for winter storage at the yacht club, I found that the hull had changed shape sufficiently for all of the new engine mounts to be distorted again.

In the spring, with the boat back in the water, I double-checked the alignment and made adjustments until I was satisfied that things were as they should be. Every spring from now on, it's going to be on my re-commissioning checklist to ensure that the drive train is aligned and all nuts and bolts around the engine are tight. I'll also be checking that everything connected to the engine is in good order, which I should have been doing all along with the old engine.

I've added these engine-related items to my pre-cruise and in-cruise check lists – these lists are the only way I've found to avoid forgetting anything important.

THE FIRST START

The engine test start was finally made at the end of the summer – the project had taken much longer than I had expected, especially with all the little things that needed to be done to completely finish it. I thought they would take a week but they actually took a month worth of weekends and quite often after work.

In the end it was all more or less in place, even if the starting battery was only connected with jumper cables and we had not tightened the shaft coupling bolts with a torque wrench, as required by the manual.

Fortunately, my Norwegian long-distance cruising friend, Jarle Karlsud, came to help with the engine start. Jarle has worked on engines a lot, and has a level of confidence that I lack.

We filled the tank and primary filter with diesel, turned the key, pushed the button and the engine started on the first go; but after I turned it off, it wouldn't start again. It must have started on the diesel left in the secondary filter and fuel lines from the test run at the factory.

I had wondered how the fuel was going to get from the tank to the engine on the first start, with empty fuel hoses. We filled the primary filter again and worked the manual priming lever on the engine fuel pump, but with no success.

Later I was advised to turn the engine by the crankshaft pulley to bring the cam that lifts the fuel pump push rod to the correct place. I had tried turning the engine over that way, but couldn't make it work, so we cranked it over on the starter motor.

Usually, it's enough to start the engine and then let its pump fill the fuel system from the tank, but if you have never done anything like this, the procedure isn't immediately obvious. We worked it out however, and after half an hour the engine started and settled to a healthy, reassuring diesel rumble. Phew – cheers and back-slapping!

While we were using the starter motor to fill the fuel system, we kept the seacock of the raw water intake scoop closed to ensure that, with no high-pressure exhaust gas to pump it out, the water lock of the exhaust system would not fill with water and back-flood the engine. I've since been advised that any time you're going run a cooling system like this, it's important to pack the case of the raw water

pump with gritless hand cleaner or some other water soluble gel that will lubricate the impeller, but dissolve when water starts running. Oh – and yes, we did remember to open the seacock when the engine finally started up again. Miracles do happen!

RUNNING IN THE ENGINE

For the first 50 hours a diesel engine should be operated at no more than three quarter of its recommended maximum speed. For my engine the maximum was 3,600 rpm (revolutions per minute), so the maximum running in/breaking in speed was 2,700 rpm; no problem as Vetus recommends 2,600 rpm as the cruising speed for my M3.28 engine.

A running in/breaking in period allows the pistons, cylinders, bearings and other parts to move against each other at moderate pressures and loads, while microscopic imperfections are worn away without damaging the surrounding surfaces. To help this smoothing and polishing process, it's important to vary the engine speed while frequently running in/breaking in a new engine.

With the running in/breaking in period complete, it was time to replace the engine oil and filters, adjust the valve clearances, and tighten all nuts and bolts. I had a strong magnet (by Filter Mag) on the oil filter canister, and it probably played its biggest role during the running in/breaking in period when a lot of metallic particles were generated by the pistons and other moving parts.

Some people say that it's best to use conventional mineral oil rather than synthetic oil during the running-in period, so that the small increase in friction improves the internal smoothing/polishing process, but I used the recommended synthetic oil, with satisfactory results.

For the first two hours of engine operation we kept the boat tied in its slip, ran the engine at moderate speeds, and engaged the gears to induce load. It's important in this and all engine operations to let the engine reach full temperature before shutting it down, to prevent carbon build-up from incomplete combustion on the piston tops, valves, cylinder heads, etc. Normal operating temperatures for most marine diesels range from 74° C to 91° C/165° F to 195° F.

PROBLEMS

We soon noticed that the engine speed was unstable, and on the first sea trial just off the yacht club dock it varied wildly, dropping for five to ten seconds and then picking back up. We described these symptoms to a more knowledgeable friend and he told us that air was getting into the fuel system.

Sure enough, after we'd checked every screw, nut, bolt, and all the hose clamps, we found that the US-made fuel filter/water separator had different threads from the hose nipples I'd bought locally and these connections were leaking air. Luckily, I had bought some other hose nipples at a clearance sale and they were a perfect fit, confirming the old mechanic's adage that you shouldn't throw anything away – it might come in handy someday. Many homes, garages, workshops and closets are bursting at the seams from similarly flawed logic, but we're only discussing boats in this book.

After wrapping the threaded ends of the hose nipples with Teflon tape and reconnecting the fuel hoses to the filter, the engine ran like clockwork! We didn't need to bleed air, as used to be the standard procedure after opening the fuel system on a diesel, because the Vetus, like most modern engine with a fuel return from each injector, is self-bleeding. Read the manual for your engine to determine if it's self-bleeding.

For most of the running in/breaking in period *Roobarb* was either in her slip or motoring close to home, but a couple of times we ventured further, and also tried out her new suit of sails.

My intention is to be the very model of a modern master mariner with this expensive new engine of mine, operating and maintaining it by the book, buying the best motor oil, the cleanest fuel and the highest quality filters. Even in Sweden, a veritable if somewhat chilly boating paradise, fuel docks occasionally deliver dirty and waterlogged fuel, so eternal vigilance is essential. To summarize: I will read the engine manual and do what it says!

MEASURING ENGINE SPEED

Unless your boat has a folding or feathering propeller, when you're sailing with the engine turned off a fixed-blade prop wants to windmill, effectively trying to turn the shaft and inner workings of the gearbox as though forward gear is engaged.

You can buy a shaft brake to stop this motion, but most marine transmission manufacturers, including ZF and Twin Disk Technodrive, whose gearboxes are used by Vetus, claim that their mechanical gearboxes can be left in reverse gear to lock the shaft while sailing, without damage to the gearbox.

Lubrication problems and internal damage will occur if the prop is allowed to windmill with the gears in neutral. Most of the larger hydraulic gearboxes are not damaged by being left in neutral while the prop windmills but as with all things nautical, read your manual carefully on this point. When the whole installation was completed, I had to calibrate the tachometer (engine speed gauge), which had not been connected to this engine before and, as is normal, was a few hundred revolutions per minute off. There is an adjustment screw on the back of the tachometer, but you need an independent measurement of the engine speed to make the calibration.

You may be able to borrow an electronic rev counter from your engine dealer but, if not, laser devices are available from several companies, and are cheap and simple to use. You stick a piece of reflective tape on the crankshaft pulley, point the laser beam at it, and the meter shows the number of revolutions per minute at which the engine is turning. With the engine still running, you set the tach to the speed on the laser meter.

SPECIAL TOOLS

The jig was a great help in adapting the engine bed for the new engine – I don't know how I'd have managed without it. Many dealers will lend you a jig when you buy an engine, and if the engine bed needs to be altered a lot, which is not always the case, it's a great advantage to be able to borrow the jig several times after the initial mark-up, as you cut and fit to get the bed just right. Don't expect to keep a borrowed jig for the duration of the project many other people will also be waiting to use it. Of course, the ultimate test device for your work on the engine bed is the engine itself, but as you can lift the jig with one hand, it make sense to get as close to perfection as you can before wrestling with a 300 pound chunk of cast iron.

Before you start using the jig, double check all of its dimensions against the actual engine – products change, jigs get mislabeled and Murphy's Law is always in full force and effect on boat work. I was so concerned about getting the engine mounts in the right place, without their rubber cores being distorted while at rest, that after all the work with the jig I put the engine in, made a rough alignment, eased the load off the mounts to allow them to straighten, and then used the actual holes in the base plates of the mounts as my drill pattern for the holes in the bed irons. After all of that, I took the engine back out before drilling the holes and tapping threads into them. You can read more about getting the engine mounts right in the previous chapter of this book.

I lifted the engine in and out three times during the project, both to check my calculations and to gain access to the engine space so that I could install other new equipment.

EXPERIENCE GAINED, INSIGHT TO SHARE

If you, like me, have no previous experience of working with engines and are, at best, average at practical things you're going to spend a long time in the boat to do a similar repower project, and depending on your location, that may be in the cold winter months, so that you'll have the boat ready for the sailing season. I photograph or film all of my boat work, and frequently dismantle completed assemblies to pose their elements for different and more illuminating views, all of which takes time.

Discounting this 'non-productive' time, I estimate that I spent 250–300 hours working on this repowering project, which included not just changing the engine but also many related sub-projects such as installing tanks, assembling a fire suppression system, soundproofing the engine enclosure and many, many, other small but necessary jobs that took a lot longer than I expected.

I spent a lot of time thinking about how best to install the equipment in the very confined space available for it on *Roobarb*, a reality for most repower projects on recreational boats, especially sailboats, where the designers think about engines as auxiliary sources of power and allocate space accordingly.

As long as the project took, the guidance and help of my professional friends probably cut the time in half and I thank them all. If you're going to have a

go at a repower project, get the help of at least one industry professional. But, if, heaven forbid, I should ever have to do it again, the job would go much faster – but of course, that's the point of experience, you've already made the mistakes.

One of the most enjoyable aspects of this project was the quiet time spent with pencil and sketch pad, dreaming and drawing. There's probably a bit of an inventor and designer in all of us, just waiting for a project boat to come along.

ESTIMATED AND ACTUAL TIME

Everything takes longer that you think it's going to, so expect obstacles and expect that any item you need immediately will not be in stock and will have to be ordered.

Everything also takes longer when spring approaches and all the boatyards and craftsmen are busy getting everyone else's boats ready for the season. I started at the end of February intending to be finished by the beginning of the summer, but to accomplish that, I would have had to remove the old engine and clean out the engine space by the end of January. I should have taken out the old engine out before the boat was hauled in September, using the dockside crane to lift out the old engine and put it on a pallet or into a trailer.

That would have saved a lot of time, but as my American friend John says, 'woulda, coulda, shoulda, but didn't'.

In the autumn, before the cold weather set in, I could have laminated the fibreglass of the new engine bed and applied the two-part bilge paint that needed temperatures above 10° C/50° F to harden well.

In the middle of a cold Swedish winter you can only work for a couple of hours at a stretch, unless you've got the boat in a heated space.

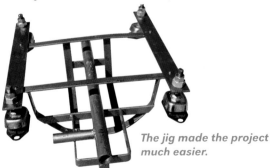

The jig made the project much easier.

SUMMARY OF COSTS

Engine (Vetus 3.28) with gearbox, engine mounts and panel, retail price*	£5,300
Propeller	£249
Shaft	£180
Flexible shaft coupling	£273
Shaft seal	£142
Steel bars for engine bed	£38
Engine controls	£190
Fuel tank level sensor	£36
No-smell filter for fuel tank breather hose,.	£80
Fuel tank breather nipple	£17
Tanks (total 240 l)	£539
Deck fill fitting for diesel fuel	£49
Tank connection kit with modifications	£173
Raw water strainer	£83
Water lock muffler	£118
Gooseneck	£95
Vacuum-breaking air vent	£82
Transom exhaust outlet	£24
Exhaust hose	£106
Miscellaneous (hose clamps, epoxy, glass fibre cloth, etc.)	£77
Sub Total for engine installation exc. VAT	**£7,851**

Bilge pumps (6 pieces)	£414
Bilge water hoses (8 metre, 38 mm diameter and 5 m, 25 mm diameter)	£144
Bilge water/oil separating filter	£86
Bilge water discharge skin fitting/through-hull (Delrin)	£5
Starting battery	£212
Battery cables	£135
Fire extinguisher (powder)	£48
Fire port	£20
Paint for engine room including brushes, etc.	£67
Fiberglass kit (epoxy resin + strips of glassfibre combination cloth)	£500
Light for the engine room	£48
Acoustic insulation	£144
Miscellaneous (hose clamps, etc.)	£76
Sub total for 'around the engine' equipment exc. VAT	**£1,899**
Grand total, exc. VAT	**£9,750**
(including 20% UK VAT)	**£11,700**

These are retail list prices with the price for the new Vetus M3.28 engine that has replaced the M3.09 that I bought. It is sometimes possible to find engines at reduced prices at boat shows. Roobarb's engine was a display model and a bit cheaper than list price.

Micke's top 5 tips

1 Get started in the autumn by taking out the old engine then cleaning and painting the bilge, etc.
2 Replace all surrounding and related systems. It's a relatively small cost when you are already doing the job.
3 Get help from an expert if you feel unsure about how to proceed, especially if it's related to the engine bed changes and alignment.
4 Measure twice – cut once!
5 Don't underestimate how long it will take to change an engine, allow time for the odd delay.

FOCUS # LESSONS LEARNED, KNOWLEDGE GAINED

1 CHOICE OF ENGINE

The torque, gearbox reduction ratio and fuel consumption of the new engine were not significant issues in my selection process. Making a minutely detailed comparison of the technical and performance characteristics of the available engines became less important to me than selecting an engine that would fit the space, and buying it from a dealer who would commit to providing help and support throughout the installation and commissioning process.

Being able to ask frequent questions of an experienced engine professional, who would lend me a jig, was the deciding factor in my choice of engine.

2 COSTS

My fretting about the financial pluses and minuses of each engine, trying to balance low base costs with high costs for spare parts and maintenance items, proved to have been unnecessary, although there can be substantial price differences between manufacturers – it's a moving market. It makes good sense to check the cost of service/maintenance parts (impeller, oil/fuel filter elements and drive belts), as the cost differs a lot from brand to brand of engine.

3 THE SCOPE OF THE PROJECT

I ended up doing far more than originally planned, as it came to light that additional items needed replacement, which would be much harder to get to and action, if I postponed them until after the basic project was complete and access was blocked or reduced by the new engine.

I replaced just about everything related to the engine, from the propeller shaft to the electrical system, but I'm convinced that it was worth it, as I'm now confident that the boat's drive train will not let me down in an emergency at sea.

My planned schedule – to have the project completed in ten weeks – proved to be unrealistic. I should have done thorough research on all aspects of the job a year in advance, then removed the old engine as soon as the boat was hauled out for the winter, and immediately re-built the engine bed and painted the engine enclosure and bilge before it got too cold for such work. With those temperature-sensitive things done, I could have finished all the other sub-systems during the winter and installed the engine in the early Spring, immediately after the boat show at which I bought the new engine.

When the engine was in, the many small jobs that still needed to be done consumed a lot of time. If you're planning a repower project for your boat, I recommend that you allow a month in the schedule, after engine installation, to complete the project, so that you're ready for the boating season without a last minute panic.

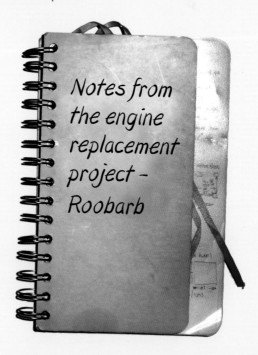

Notes from the engine replacement project – Roobarb

>> STEP-BY-STEP

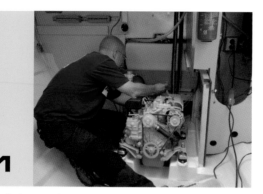

1

▲ All the small jobs at the end were very time consuming and I worked every day to get them finished in time to get some sailing in before the season was over.

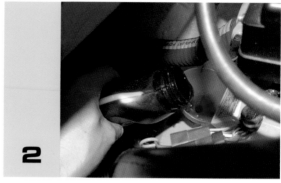

2

▲ Fluids had to be topped up in several places and, to avoid missing anything, I checked the manual carefully for the correct fill locations and levels.

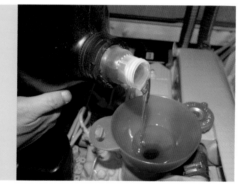

3

▲ Oil in the gearbox and the engine sump/pan was added in accordance with the instruction booklet. I checked and double checked the levels.

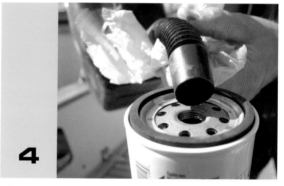

4

▲ The fuel filter and hoses were filled with diesel before the first engine start. It started on the first turn of the key.

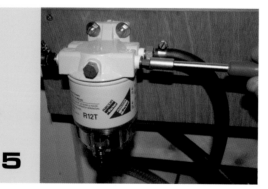

5

▲ The fuel system was taking in air. We finally found the problem in the primary filter hose connections, which needed hose nipples with the correct thread.

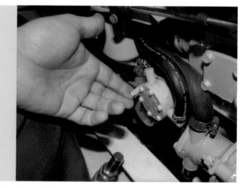

6

▲ We had problems starting the engine again and tried to pump diesel with the priming lever on the fuel pump. By cranking the engine over on the starter motor. We finally got the fuel to circulate.

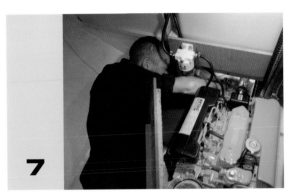

▲ With Jarle's help, I tightened the bolts on the shaft coupling to the correct torque.

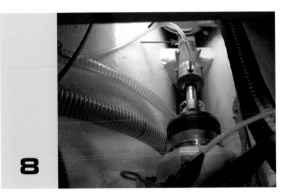

▲ We checked the systems surrounding the engine and made several adjustments. Here you can see the oil level in the hose of the shaft seal.

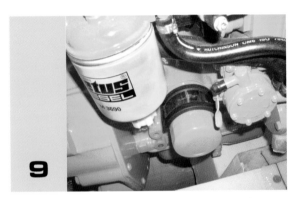

▲ I added a purpose-made magnet to the oil filter and it collected a surprising quantity of metal particles during the running in/breaking in period.

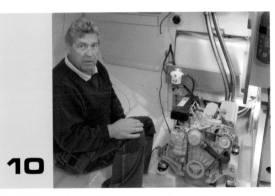

▲ With the help of my expert adviser, Bo Linderholm, all important systems were checked. Bo also gave me some welcome ideas about making improvements to what I'd done.

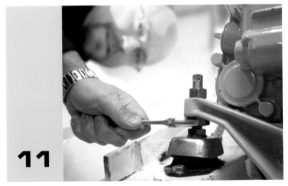

▲ Bo used a spanner/open-ended wrench to double check, by feel, that the engine was bearing equally on all four mounts.

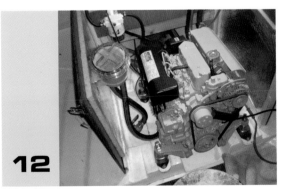

▲ Bo gave the thumbs up and the engine was ready for a test start.

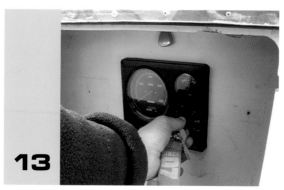

▲ After letting the glow plugs heat up for six seconds, I turned the key and it started right up.

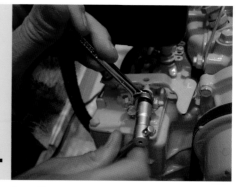

▲ Using the adjustment screw on the high-pressure injection pump, I set the idling speed to 800 rpm.

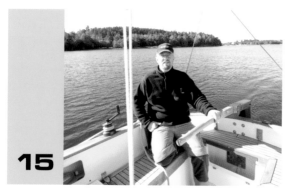

▲ Some days later I was out 'for real' for the first time after a couple of short sea trials. The new engine obediently idled along at low speed. Project ending!

PROJECT LOG 🔧🔧🔧

LEVEL OF DIFFICULTY: medium

TIME SPENT: 30 hours.

TOOLS: Large spanners/open ended wrenches, laser tachometer, torque wrench.

CHECKING/ADJUSTING VALVE CLEARANCE

When the engine has done its first 50 hours and the running-in/breaking-in process was finished, the valve clearances need to be checked. This isn't a difficult job and if you managed to install the engine yourself, you can certainly check and adjust the valves. Here's the process I followed on *Roobarb*'s new engine.

Checking the valve clearance must be done with a cold engine, ie one that has not been run for at least six hours. Remove the rocker cover from the engine cylinder head to expose the valve stems, valve springs, rocker arms, rocker shaft, tappets, push rods and many other somewhat intimidating bits of complicated machinery. Take the rocker cover off carefully to avoid damaging the gasket between the rocker cover and the cylinder head. Even though you'll probably end up installing a new gasket, unless you had the foresight to

order one before starting this job, the old one will keep you going until the new gasket arrives. Bring piston number one to top dead centre of its compression stroke by turning the engine over with a breaker bar or other long handle moving a socket on the crankshaft pulley bolt until the TDC marks on the engine block and crankshaft pulley are lined up. These marks are illustrated in the engine's service manual.

Note: there are two TDCs in a four-stroke engine cycle; one as the piston comes up to compress the air in the cylinder, the other as the same piston comes back up to force the products of combustion out of the cylinder after the downwards power stroke. At TDC of the compression stroke, the inlet and exhaust valves are both closed, and the rocker arms for this cylinder will not move when the crankshaft is turned a little – the gaps between the rocker arm and the tappets are open. Start with cylinder number one, the one closest to the front of the engine (the end where the crankshaft pulley, alternator, drive belt etc. are located). With that piston at compression TDC, you should be able to just insert the 0.25mm /0.10" blade of a feeler gauge into the gaps between the rocker arm ends and the tappet heads of the two valves for cylinder number one. If the gap is too large or too small, use a spanner/open ended wrench to back off the tappet locknut, adjust the tappet up or down with a flat-head screwdriver engaged in the top slot of the tappet, then holding the tappet still with the screwdriver, retighten the lock nut.

This is a fiddly little process, so have a set of tappets and locknuts on hand for when you strip a thread and don't get exasperated when it takes a few attempts for you get the hang of it.

Now turn the crankshaft 240° clockwise and repeat the process for cylinder number 3, then turn another 240° and repeat for cylinder number 2. Carefully inspect the whole area of the cylinder head, to make sure you haven't left anything behind (a nut, a washer, a screwdriver bit, etc.) then replace the rocker cover, with its new gasket. Valve clearances for the Vetus M3.28 are set at 0.25mm/0.10", but read your engine service manual both for the recommended valve clearances, and possible variations on this process. Checking valve clearance should be done every 500 operating hours of the engine – or every year according to most instruction books. The recommendation is somewhat strict, but at least do it every other year rather than not doing it at all.

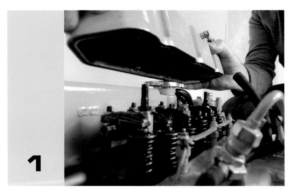

▲ Remove the two nuts of the rocker cover to get access to the valves.

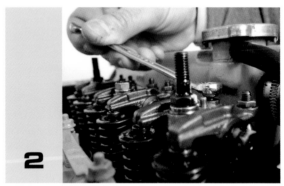

▲ Loosen the lock nut on the tappet of valve one.

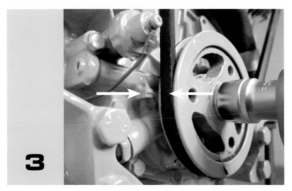

▲ Identify the TDC mark on the crank pulley to be aligned clockwise with the mark on the engine block.

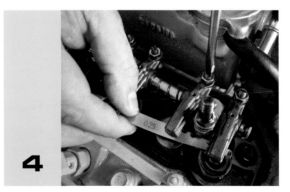

▲ Check the valve lash (clearance) with a feeler gauge.

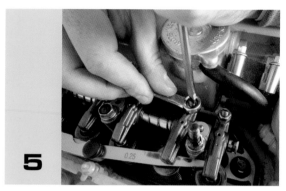

5

▲ Adjust lash (clearance) with a flat screwdriver and spanner/open ended wrench if necessary.

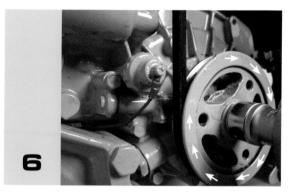

6

▲ Turn the crank pulley 240° clockwise with the help of a spanner. Then repeat this procedure for next cylinder.

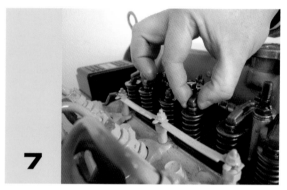

7

▲ You can check if you reached the TDC – the rocker should be slightly loose. Use the bar and socket on the crankshaft nut to turn the crankshaft a little to get the correct position.

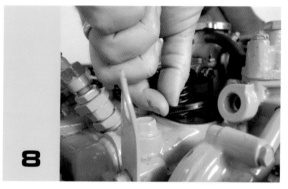

8

▲ Use new gasket for the rocker cover as it will otherwise leak oil sooner or later.

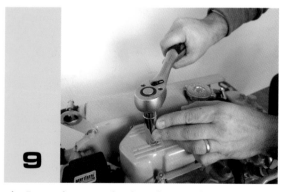

9

▲ Put rocker cover back and reattach the hoses.

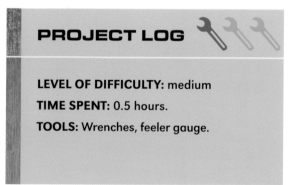

PROJECT LOG

LEVEL OF DIFFICULTY: medium

TIME SPENT: 0.5 hours.

TOOLS: Wrenches, feeler gauge.

FOCUS WARRANTY

Laws and regulations related to warranties and consumer protection vary from country to country. Most countries impose a minimum warranty period for various product categories but many manufacturers, as a demonstration of confidence in the quality of their products, provide longer warranties as a part of the standard package.

Even if you install the engine yourself, your country's laws will most likely protect you from manufacturing defects providing you report any problems to the manufacturer, in writing and within the warranty period.

After talking to several engine dealers, I came to the conclusion that there is no common practice as to how marine engine warranties are honored and claims processed.

In most cases, if you buy the engine direct from a dealer, the warranty period starts on the day that you take delivery but if you buy it through an installer approved by the manufacturer, the warranty period usually starts on the day the installation is completed. For do-it-yourself installers, who may complete the installation many months after buying the engine, or for boat owners who have their engines professionally installed during the Autumn, several months of the warranty period may have passed before the engine is used.

This leads to another unintended consequence where engine buyers take delivery at the last minute, which is not in the interests of the installers or the manufacturers as it bunches shipments and installations into a short period of the spring and early summer, creating supply chain spikes and dips, scheduling difficulties and over-stretched support services, all leading to unhappy boat owners.

Be sure to check the terms of your engine warranty so that you understand when the warranty period will start and end. Also ask if the purchase price includes a pre-start inspection of your do-it-yourself installation by a qualified professional. If such an inspection is not included in the base price, negotiate for one with the salesman before you buy the engine. As with every other part of life, there is nothing free when it comes to what people do to earn a living, so be realistic, one way or another you're going to pay for a pre-start inspection, but however it occurs, it will be the best money you've ever spent on your boat – insurance the possibility of an engine-destroying mistake in the cooling and exhaust systems.

The warranty from Vetus, as with a few other manufacturers, is valid for three years after a first start that takes place within a year of the initial delivery, and the warranty is extended to five years for some parts of the engine such as the block. Vetus, too, requires the authorized dealer that sold the engine to formally inspect and sign-off on the installation.

Diesel Power AB, who sell Solé in Sweden, trust the client to do a good job and do not require a pre-start inspection, but do inspect if a claim is made on the warranty. Once again, you have to be realistic – a manufacturer's warranty will not cover damage resulting from installation mistakes, from misuse or a lack of maintenance and appropriate care.

When buying a new engine, negotiate in the price of the engine to include installation support for you – that you can phone an engineer and ask for advice about the installation. This is also in the manufacturer's best interests, as it reduces the incidence of claims and disagreements. It's very important to discuss and understand the level of support available to you as a do-it-yourself engine installer before buying an engine and embarking on a repower project.

This is what Michael An, Director of Sales for Vetus in Sweden had to say about it:

'If the authorized dealer who sold the engine can come and do an inspection, and certify that the installation has been carried out properly, the warranty starts on the day of the first test run of the engine'.

Michael also thinks that the buyer should be sensible and not buy an engine in Edinburgh to install in Bristol – in order to save a few quid, and then expect the sales rep to swing by the boat for a chat on a regular basis.

Björn Sjöberg at Sjöbergs Marine, who sells Yanmar and Beta engines, says:

'If the installation is correct, there will be no problem with the warranty – that starts from the time you fill in the warranty card'.

It's not that often that there are serious problems with do-it-yourself engine installations but as I've emphasized in previous chapters, if the engine is flooded with water as a result of an improperly designed and installed exhaust system or cooling system, perhaps with an undersized water lock or missing air vent, the ensuing and very expensive damage will not be covered by any manufacturer's warranty. If you want to be sure that you're completely covered, you need to thoroughly discuss and understand the terms and condition of the warranty, especially with regard to start dates, coverage periods and inspection requirements. Negotiate any additional coverage that you want before you sign the purchase agreement, but remember that in general you can't insure yourself against your own negligence, lack of preparedness and misconduct – those are legal more than engine insurance issues, and are the subject of several other very good books.

loss of profits, haul-out fees, launch, towing, storage, slip fees, insurance coverage, loan payment, transportation fees, telephone charges and mileage. The limitations in this Limited Warranty apply regardless of whether your claims are based on breach of contract, tort (including negligence and strict liability) or any other theory. Any action arising hereunder must be brought within (1) year after the cause of action accrues or it shall be barred. Some states and countries do not allow certain limitations on warranties or for breach of warranties. Limitations set forth in this paragraph shall not apply to the extent that they are prohibited by law.

Purchaser's Responsibility and Items Excluded from Warranty

- Performing regular maintenance and the costs associated with regular maintenance, specified in the applicable Operation Manual;
- Mantaining records of all recommended service and maintenance;
- Ordinary wear and tear;
- Any YANMAR Marine Product, accessory or part that has been, in YANMAR's sole judgment, subject to negligence, misuse, accident, improper installation, improper maintenance, racing or engaging in a contest of speed or endurance, use of non approved attachments or non genuine parts, unreasonable exposure to the environment or serviced by an unauthorized facility;
- Cost associated with consumable parts;
- Cost of transporting the YANMAR Marine Product, part or the vessel in which such YANMAR Marine Product(s) are installed to and from the service facility designated by YANMAR for warranty repair;
- Consequence of any modification or alteration of a YANMAR Marine Product or part from which the serial number has been removed, altered or otherwise tampered with;

6 www.yanmarmarine.com

An example (from Yanmar) of the text in the manual on the warranty.

09

REFERENCES

Tools and equipment

Replacing the engine in a small recreational boat does not require many special tools – the equipment already in your toolbox will do for most of the work. Having said that, here are some slightly unusual items that I suggest you obtain before starting a repower project – they'll make the job a lot easier. I've described how and when they are used.

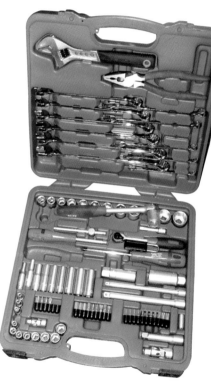

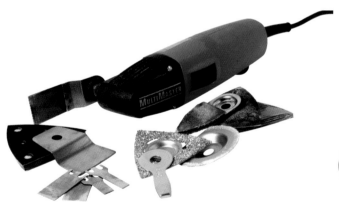

The Multimaster (also in other brands) is an oscillating tool that is fitted with different blades and pads to saw, cut, shape or sand just about anything, in the tightest of spots and with very little dust or mess.

Rigged as a saw it makes very fine cuts in places where other saws just won't fit and is ideal for plunge (straight-down) cuts in wood and fibreglass.

A full set of tools of good quality, like this set from Kanasa makes life so much simpler.

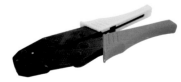

An electrician's ratchet crimper is the only way to go for crimp connections, which are also the only way to go for connecting electrical wires on a boat. Standard pliers and other squeezing and gripping tools just won't do the job properly.

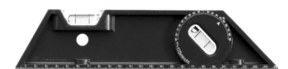

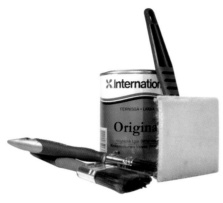

A spirit level with an adjustable bubble, used in combination with the engine jig, was indispensible. I wouldn't have wanted to be without either of them on this job. A wide range of spirit levels is available, but the simplest, costing less than £20/$30, worked perfectly.

The highest quality brushes, pads and rollers are essential for getting a satisfactory finish with marine grade paints, although rolling on its own should be enough for out-of-sight places like the engine compartment. Never forget that good results come from meticulous preparation of the surfaces to be painted; the quality of the brushes won't make much difference if you haven't prepared well.

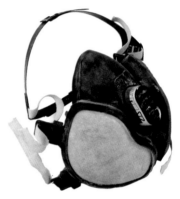

It may be possible to lift an engine by the mainsheet or a vang tackle attached to the boom but an inexpensive chain hoist, sometimes called a chain fall, makes the job a lot easier and doesn't strain your boom and blocks. Chain hoists are available in DIY stores and from tool catalogues.

If you use two-part paint in the engine compartment or re-work the engine bed with fibreglass lamination of any resin type, a good respirator is essential. It's best to use a closed mask with a forced air supply, but nothing less than a half mask with a filter rated for fine particles and organic solvent vapor will be adequate here.

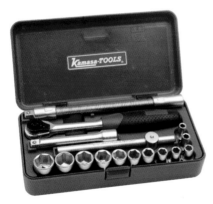

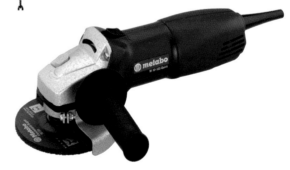

A socket set with a ratchet handle, breaker bar and extension bars is a must if you don't already have one in your toolbox. The nuts and bolts on most European engines are all metric, but some older engines and some US-built engines have Imperial fasteners, so check this before you buy new sockets, spanners and wrenches.

An angle grinder with a bronze or plastic (not steel) wire brush can be effective in removing engrained surface dirt. This grinder, with an appropriate disk, can also be used to cut the flat irons for the engine bed and many other hard objects.

ENGINE GUIDE

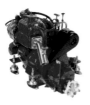 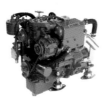 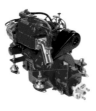 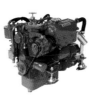

Manufacturer	Beta Marin	Beta Marin	Beta Marin	Beta Marin
Model	Beta 14	Beta 16	Beta 20	Beta25
Number of cylinders	2	2	3	3
Cylinder - bore x stroke	67 x 68	72 x 73,6	57 x 68	72 x 73,6
Total displacement in litres	478	599	719	898
Flywheel power (hp/kW)	13,3/9,94	16,7/11,7	20/14,4	24,8/18,15
Max speed (rpm)	3600	3600	3600	3600
Torque/engine speed (Nm/rpm)	32/2600	32/2600	46/2600	55/2600
Compression ratio	23:1	23:1	23:1	23:1
Fuel injection method	Indirect injection	Indirect injection	Indirect injection	Indirect injection
Dry weight with gearbox-kg/lbs	89/196	93/205	102/225	118/260
Cooling system	Fresh water cooling	Fresh water cooling	Fresh water cooling	Fresh water cooling
Block manufacturer	Kubota	Kubota	Kubota	Kubota
Generator output – amps/volts	40	40	40	40
Max installation angle – long axis	15	15	15	15
Standard gearbox	TMC40	TMC40	TMC40	TMC40
Standard reduction ratio	2,0-2,6	2,0-2,6	2,0-2,6	2,0-2,6
Dimensions (L x W x H in mm)	583x430x582	597x427x562	655x428x583	678x427x562
General agent in the UK	Beta Marine, www. betamarine.co.uk	Beta Marine, www. betamarine.co.uk	Beta Marine, www. betamarine.co.uk	Beta Marine, www. betamarine.co.uk

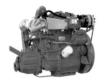

Manufacturer	Beta Marin	Beta Marin	Bukh	Bukh
Model	Beta 35	Beta 38	DV24ME	DV32ME
Number of cylinders	4	4	2	2
Cylinder - bore x stroke	76 x 73,6	78 x 78,4	85/85	85/85
Total displacement in litres	1335	1498	964	964
Flywheel power (hp/kW)	35/25,7	37,5/27,6	24/17,6	32/23,5
Max speed (rpm)	3600	3000	3600	3600
Torque/engine speed (Nm/rpm)	86/2600	90/2200	55/1800	70/2400
Compression ratio	22:1	22:1	–	–
Fuel injection method	Indirect injection	Indirect injection	Injection pump	Injection pump
Dry weight with gearbox-kg/lbs	170/375	170/375	210/463	218/509
Cooling system	Fresh water cooling	Fresh water cooling	Direct seawater	Direct seawater
Block manufacturer	Kubota	Kubota	Bukh	Bukh
Generator output – amps/volts	65	65	50	50
Max installation angle – long axis	15	15	12	12
Standard gearbox	PRM80	PRM120	ZF	ZF
Standard reduction ratio	2,04-2,6	2,04-2,5-2,94	3:1	3:1 2,5:1 2:1
Dimensions (L x W x H in mm)	867 x 504 x 625	888 x 504 x 625	845 x 470 x 640	845 x 470 x 640
General agent in the UK	Beta Marine, www.betamarine.co.uk	Beta Marine, www.betamarine.co.uk	Bukh Diesel UK Ltd, www.bukh.co.uk	Bukh Diesel UK Ltd, www.bukh.co.uk

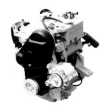

Bukh	Bukh	Iveco	Iveco	Iveco
DV36ME	DV48ME	4021 M20	4031 M30	4041 M40
3	3	2	3	4
85/85	85/85	75 x 77,6	75 x 77,6	75 x 77,6
1447	1447	686	1028	1372
3928.7	48	20/14,7	30/22,1	40/29,4
3600	35.8	3600	3600	3600
90/1800	100/3000	44,5/2200	64/2000	87/2400
-	-	22,8:1	22,8:1	22,8:1
Injection pump	Injection pump	Indirect injection	Indirect injection	Indirect injection
265/584	273/602	99/218	115/254	133/293
Direct seawater	Direct seawater	Fresh water cooling	Fresh water cooling	Fresh water cooling
Bukh	Bukh	Lombardini	Lombardini	Lombardini
50	50	65	65	65
15	15	15	15	10
ZF	ZF	TMC40	TMC40	TMC40
3:1	2:1	2:1 alt. 2,6:1	2:1 alt. 2,6:1	2:1 alt. 2,6:1
928 x 535 x 634	928 x 535 x 676	560 x 488 x 522	643 x 488 x 452	726 x 488 x 549
Bukh Diesel UK Ltd, www.bukh.co.uk	Bukh Diesel UK Ltd, www.bukh.co.uk	Powertrain Technologies, www. ivecomotors.com	Powertrain Technologies, www. ivecomotors.com	Powertrain Technologies, www. ivecomotors.com

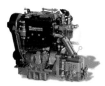   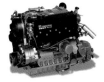

Manufacturer	Lombardini	Lombardini	Lombardini	Lombardini
Model	LDW 502 M	LDW 702 M	LDW 1003 M	LDW 1404 M
Number of cylinders	2	2	3	4
Cylinder - bore x stroke	72 x 62	75 x 77,6	75 x 77,6	75 x77,6
Total displacement in litres	505	686	1028	1372
Flywheel power (hp/kW)	13/9,5	20/14,7	30/22,1	40/29,4
Max speed (rpm)	3600	3600	3600	3600
Torque/engine speed (Nm/rpm)	25,5/2200	40,5/2100	64/2200	82,5/2400
Compression ratio	22,3:1	22,8:1	22,8:1	22,8:1
Fuel injection method	Indirect injection	Indirect injection	Indirect injection	Indirect injection
Dry weight with gearbox-kg/lbs	82/181	99/218	115/254	133/293
Cooling system	Fresh water cooling	Fresh water cooling	Fresh water cooling	Fresh water cooling
Block manufacturer	Lombardini	Lombardini	Lombardini	Lombardini
Generator output – amps/volts	40	80	80	80
Max installation angle – long axis	20	20	20	20
Standard gearbox	TMC40	TMC40	TMC40	TMC40
Standard reduction ratio	1,5:1, 2,0:1 alt. 2,6:1	1,5:1, 2,0:1 alt. 2,6:1	1,5:1, 2,0:1 alt. 2,6:1	1,5:1, 2,0:1 alt. 2,6:1
Dimensions (L x W x H in mm)	560 x 452 x 492	560 x 488 x 522	643 x 488 x 522	726 x 488 x 549
General agent in the UK	Salterns Marina Ltd, www.goldenarrow.co.uk	Salterns Marina Ltd, www.goldenarrow.co.uk	Salterns Marina Ltd, www.goldenarrow.co.uk	Salterns Marina Ltd, www.goldenarrow.co.uk

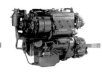 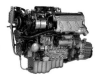

Nanni	Nanni	Nanni	Nanni	Nanni
N2.10	N 2.14	N 3.21	N 3.30	N 4.38
2	2	3	3	4
67 x 68	67 x 68	67 x 68	78 x 78,4	78 x 78,4
479	479	719	1231	1498
10/7,36	14/10.3	21/15,4	29/21,3	37,5/27,6
3000	3600	3600	3600	3000
26/2200	30/2600	45/2600	65/2600	110/2200
23:1	23:1	23:1	23:1	22:1
Indirect injection	Indirect injection	Indirect injection	Indirect injection	pre-combustion chamber
87/192	92/203	105/231	145/320	145/320
Fresh water cooling	Fresh water cooling	Fresh water cooling	Fresh water cooling	Fresh water cooling
Kubota	Kubota	Kubota	Kubota	Kubota
40	70	70	100	100
15	15	15	15	15
TMC-40	TMC-40	TMC-40	TMC-40	TMC-60
2,6:1	2.0-2.6	2.0-2.6	2.0-2.6	2.0-2.6
558 x 428 x 486	573 x 478 x 511	673,5 x 478 x 511	745 x 467 x 589	891,5 x 482 x 598
A.R. Peachment Ltd, www.peachment.co.uk	A.R. Peachment Ltd, www.peachment.co.uk	A.R. Peachment Ltd, www.peachment.co.uk	A.R. Peachment Ltd, www.peachment.co.uk	A.R. Peachment Ltd, www.peachment.co.uk

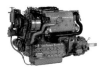

Manufacturer	Nanni	Nanni	Sole	Sole
Model	N 4.40	N 4.50	Mini-17	Mini-29
Number of cylinders	4	4	2	3
Cylinder - bore x stroke	80 x 92,4	87 x 92,4	76 x 70	76 x 70
Total displacement in litres	1857	2197	635	952
Flywheel power (hp/kW)	40/29,4	50/36,8	16/11,7	27,2/20
Max speed (rpm)	2800	2800	3600	3600
Torque/engine speed (Nm/rpm)	115/2000	160/1600	36/1500	52/2200
Compression ratio	21:1	21:1	23:1	22:1
Fuel injection method	pre-combustion chamber	pre-combustion chamber	Indirect injection	Indirect injection
Dry weight with gearbox-kg/lbs	225/496	232/511	95/209	105/231
Cooling system	Fresh water cooling	Fresh water cooling	Fresh water cooling	Fresh water cooling
Block manufacturer	Kubota	Kubota	Mitsubishi	Mitsubishi
Generator output – amps/volts	100	100	40	40
Max installation angle – long axis	15	15	20	20
Standard gearbox	TMC-60	TMC-60	TMC-40	TMC-40
Standard reduction ratio	2.0-2.6	2.0-2.6	2:1 2,6:1	2:1 2,6:1
Dimensions (L x W x H in mm)	947 x 562 x 627	965 x 562 x 627	615 x 480x503	703 x 482x532
General agent in the UK	A.R. Peachment Ltd, www.peachment.co.uk	A.R. Peachment Ltd, www.peachment.co.uk	Diamond Diesels (UK) Limited, www. solediesels.co.uk	Diamond Diesels (UK) Limited, www. solediesels.co.uk

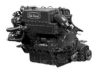 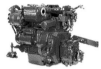

Sole	Sole	Westerbeke	Westerbeke	Westerbeke
Mini-33	Mini-44	12D	30C	35E
3	4	2	3	3
78 x 92	78 x 92	76 x 70	76 x 70	78 x 92
1318	1758	630	950	1318
31,4/23,1	42/30,9	12/9	27/20	31/23
3000	3000	3000	3600	3000
80/2000	108/1750	40,5/2200	60/2120	80/1940
22:1	22:1	23:1	23:1	22:1
Indirect injection	Indirect injection	Indirect injection	Indirect injection	Indirect injection
152/335	172/379	102/225	124/274	175/386
Fresh water cooling	Fresh water cooling	Fresh water cooling	Fresh water cooling	Fresh water cooling
Mitsubishi	Mitsubishi	Mistubushi	Mistubushi	Mistubushi
50	50	50	50	50
20	20	14	14	14
TMC-40	TTMC35P	5M	PRM80	PRM120
2:1 2,6:1	2:1 2,6:1	2,05:1	2,5:1	2,0:1
742 x 531 x 581	864 x 531 x 581	622,3x508x515,6	744x478x518	776,6x541,3x573,5
Diamond Diesels (UK) Limited, www.solediesels.co.uk	Diamond Diesels (UK) Limited, www.solediesels.co.uk	Watermota Ltd, www.watermota.co.uk	Watermota Ltd, www.watermota.co.uk	Watermota Ltd, www.watermota.co.uk

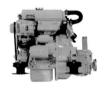   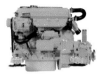

Manufacturer	VETUS	VETUS	VETUS	VETUS
Model	M2.02	M2.D5	M2.06	M3.28
Number of cylinders	2	2	2	3
Cylinder - bore x stroke	76 x 70	70 x 70	76 x 70	76 x 70
Total displacement in litres	0.635	0.538	0.635	0.952
Flywheel power (hp/kW)	12/8.8	13/9.5	16/11.8	27.2/20
Max speed (rpm)	3000	3600	3600	3600
Torque/engine speed (Nm/rpm)	28.1/3000	25/3600	29.3/3600	53.1/3600
Compression ratio	23:1	23:1	23:1	23:1
Fuel injection method	Indirect injection	Indirect injection	Indirect injection	Indirect injection
Dry weight with gearbox-kg/lbs	98/216	98/216	98/216	123/271
Cooling system	Fresh water cooling	Fresh water cooling	Fresh water cooling	Fresh water cooling
Block manufacturer	Mitsubishi	Mitsubishi	Mitsubishi	Mitsubishi
Generator output – amps/volts	75/12	75/12	75/12	75/12
Max installation angle – long axis	15	15	15	15
Standard gearbox	TMC40P	TMC40P	TMC40P	TMC40P
Standard reduction ratio	2.05/2.60:1	2.05/2.60:1	2.05/2.60:1	2.05/2.60:1
Dimensions (L x W x H in mm)	612 x 494 x 500	612 x 494x500	612 x494x500	695 x 505 x 500
General agent in the UK	Vetus Ltd, www.vetus.com	Vetus Ltd, www.vetus.com	Vetus Ltd, www.vetus.com	Vetus Ltd, www.vetus.com

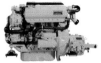   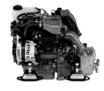

VETUS	VETUS	VETUS	Volvo	Volvo
M4.15	M4.17	M4.55	D1-13	D1-20
4	4	4	2	3
78 x 78.5	78 x 92	78 x 92	67 x 72	67 x 72
1.5	1.758	1.758	510	760
33/24.3	42/30.9	52/38.3	12,2/9	18,8/13,8
3000	3000	3000	3200	3200
77.4/3600	98/3000	127/2000	29/1600	47/2400
22:1	22:1	22:1	23,5:1	23,5:1
Indirect injection	Indirect injection	Indirect injection	Injection pump	Injection pump
180/397	185/408	192/432	113/249	131/289
Fresh water cooling	Fresh water cooling	Fresh water cooling	Fresh water cooling	Fresh water cooling
Mitsubishi	Mitsubishi	Mitsubishi	Shibaura/Perkins	Shibaura/Perkins
110/12	110/12	110/12	115	115
15	15	15	2/2800	3/2800
TMC60E	TMC60E	TMC345	MS10L/MS10A	MS10L/MS10A
2.02/2.52:1	2.02/2.52:1	2.2/2.47:1	2,35:1,2,72:1	2,35:1,2,72:1
872 x 490 x 575	872 x 490 x 575	882 x 490 x 578	651 x 476 x 514	681 x 471 x 534
Vetus Ltd, www.vetus.com	Vetus Ltd, www.vetus.com	Vetus Ltd, www.vetus.com	Volvo Penta, www.volvopenta.com	Volvo Penta, www.volvopenta.com

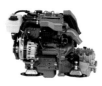   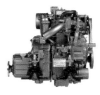

Manufacturer	Volvo	Volvo	Volvo	Yanmar
Model	D1-30	D2-40	D2-55	1GM10
Number of cylinders	3	4	4	1
Cylinder - bore x stroke	77 x 81	77 x 81	84 x 100	75 x 72
Total displacement in litres	1130	1510	1510	318
Flywheel power (hp/kW)	28,4/20,9	39,6/29,1	55/41	9/6,7
Max speed (rpm)	3200	3200	3000	3600
Torque/engine speed (Nm/rpm)	72/2200	97/2000	135/2400	18/3000
Compression ratio	23,5:1	23,5:1	23,3:1	-
Fuel injection method	Injection pump	Injection pump	Injection pump	pre-combustion chamber
Dry weight with gearbox-kg/lbs	145/320	178/392	249/549	81/179
Cooling system	Fresh water cooling	Fresh water cooling	Fresh water cooling	Direct seawater
Block manufacturer	Shibaura/Perkins	Shibaura/Perkins	Shibaura/Perkins	Yanmar
Generator output – amps/volts	115	115	115	35
Max installation angle – long axis	4,5/2800	6/2800	12/2600	1,6/3200
Standard gearbox	MS10L/MS10A	MS15A/MS15L	MS25A/MS25L	KM2P-1
Standard reduction ratio	2,35:1,2,72:1	2,14:1 2,63:1	2,29:1 2,71:1	2,21:1,262:1,322:1
Dimensions (L x W x H in mm)	728 x 482 x553	812 x 482 x 574	649 x 543,5 x 557,3	554 x 370 x 485
General agent in the UK	Volvo Penta, www.volvopenta.com	Volvo Penta, www.volvopenta.com	Volvo Penta, www.volvopenta.com	E.P. Barrus Ltd, www.yanmarmarine.co.uk

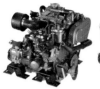 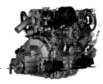 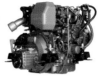

Yanmar	Yanmar	Yanmar	Yanmar
2YM15	3YM20	3YM30	3JH5-E
2	3	3	3
70 x 74	70 x 74	76 x 82	88 x 90
570	854	1115	1642
14/10,3	22/16,2	30/22,1	38,5/28,7
3600	3600	3600	3000
34/2400	51/2500	70/2500	115/1750
-	-	-	-
Indirect injection	Indirect injection	Indirect injection	Injection pump
113/249	130/287	133/293	173/381
Fresh water cooling	Fresh water cooling	Fresh water cooling	Fresh water cooling
Yanmar	Yanmar	Yanmar	Yanmar
60	60	80	80
2,5/3200	4/3200	5/3250	6,5/2750
KM2P-1	KM2P-1	KM2P-1	KM35P
2,21:1,262:1,322:1	2,21:1,262:1,322:1	2,21:1,262:1,322:1	2,36:1,2,61:1
613 x 463 x 600,3	693 x 463 x600,3	715,5 x 462 x 618	770 x 517,6 x 622,6
E.P. Barrus Ltd, www.yanmarmarine.co.uk	E.P. Barrus Ltd, www.yanmarmarine.co.uk	E.P. Barrus Ltd, www.yanmarmarine.co.uk	E.P. Barrus Ltd, www.yanmarmarine.co.uk

INDEX